Wild Plants

and

Native Peoples

of the

Four Corners

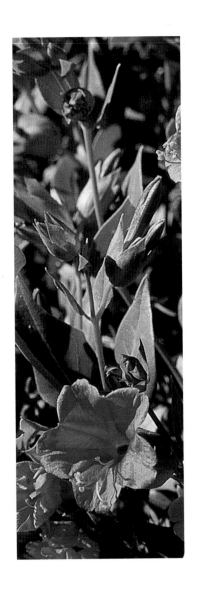

Wild
Plants

and

Native
Peoples

of the

Four
Corners

BY WILLIAM W. DUNMIRE
AND GAIL D. TIERNEY

MUSEUM OF NEW MEXICO PRESS
SANTA FE

Line-art illustrations by Gail D. Tierney
Color Photography by William W. Dunmire

Copyright © 1997 Museum of New Mexico Press. Photographs by William D. Dunmire © the photographer. *All rights reserved.* No part of this book may be reproduced in any form or by any means whatsoever without the expressed written consent of the publisher, with the exception of brief excerpts embodied in critical reviews.

Project editor: Mary Wachs
Design and production: David Skolkin
Cartography: Deborah Reade
Manufactured in Korea

Library of Congress Cataloging-in-Publication Data
Dunmire, William W.
    Wild plants and native peoples of the Four Corners / by William
W. Dunmire and Gail D. Tierney
        p.   cm.
    Includes bibliographical references and index.
    ISBN 0–89013–319–0 (pb)
    1. Indians of North America—Southwest, New—Ethnobotany.
2. Ethnobotany—Four Corners Region.   3. Plants, Useful—Four
Corners Region.   4. Wild plants, Edible—Four Corners Region.
5. Medicinal plants—Four Corners Region.   I. Tierney, Gail D.,
1935–   . II. Title.
E78.S7D76 1997
581.6'09792'59—dc21   97-2372
                                                       CIP

10 9 8 7 6 5 4 3 2

Museum of New Mexico Press
Post Office Box 2087
Santa Fe, New Mexico 87504

Cover photograph: Purple aster
Frontispiece: Four-o'clock

Contents

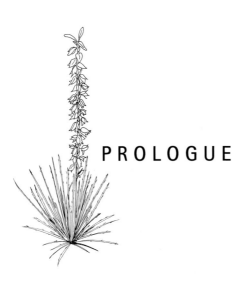

PROLOGUE

WHEN WE COMPLETED our research and writing in 1994 for *Wild Plants of the Pueblo Province*, the companion volume to this book, we realized that much remained to be said. In our first book we concentrated on the most useful plants growing within the Rio Grande River basin. We told of the people who had occupied that region during prehistoric times and of their descendants, the modern Pueblo Indians who are members of New Mexico's nineteen living pueblos.

But in order to fully chronicle the story of the modern Puebloans and their relationship with the plant world, it is necessary to shift our attention northwestward to the Four Corners, a relatively small geographical region encompassing perhaps one-eighth of the four states but of immense consequence to the developments that span the Indian Southwest. Considering this larger region allows us both to present a fuller picture of the ancient people popularly known as "Anasazi" and to include the contemporary tribes that occupy and are sus-

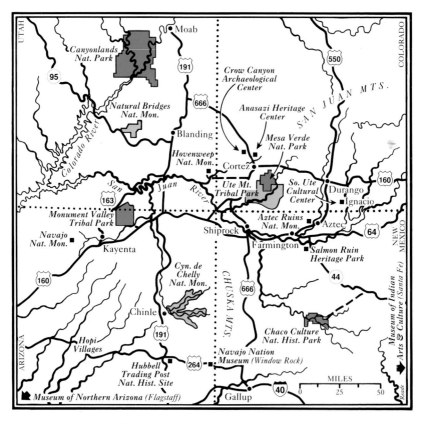

Public parks, museums, and cultural centers
in the Four Corners region.

tained by this land today: the Hopi, Navajo, Ute Mountain
Ute, and Jicarilla Apache Indians.

Wild plants have played an essential, even pivotal role in
shaping the lives of native peoples of the Four Corners
Southwest. This book explores some of the most useful wild
plants now growing in the region, with the central focus upon
the centuries-old connection between wild plants and humans
and their daily needs. For prehistoric evidence of this plant-
people relationship, we explore the flora of five different parks
within the U.S. National Park System: Chaco Culture, Aztec
Ruins, Mesa Verde, Hovenweep, and Canyon de Chelly.

Moving forward in time from the ancient dwelling sites, we arrive at the modern Hopi, who represent a direct cultural link with the pre-Puebloan people. Navajos, Utes, and Jicarilla Apaches, relative late arrivals in the region, constitute the third area of focus.

In our treatment of the many uses that these ancient and contemporary people found for wild plants we have avoided areas of plant use that might distress or offend native cultures. Thus, we do not discuss ritual plant uses, ceremonies, or other religious matters that are not meant to be shared with outsiders.

How to Use This Book

For continuity, we suggest that the first few chapters be read in sequence. Chapter 1 provides a broad overview of modern-day natural resources found in the Four Corners region. The next six chapters provide a historical overview of the region's native peoples and their practices for plant gathering and use. Chapter 8, "Weedy Gardens," examines ancestral and contemporary garden practices. Chapter 9, "Wild Plant Uses," deals directly with the multitude of uses, from food and medicine to weaving and construction. Our descriptions of such uses, as well as those contained in chapter 11, "Plants and Plantcraft," are based upon archaeological evidence, which in turn is compared with recorded uses by native people living in the region during historic times. We conclude the narrative portion of this book with a description of several techniques modern ethnobotanists use to interpret plant use.

The core of this volume features profiles of more than fifty individual plant species that have important cultural associations and are relatively easy to find growing in the Four Corners region. Using the illustrations and descriptions, the reader will be able to identify these plants in at least one of the five national parks highlighted, as well as in the field generally. While readers of *Wild Plants of the Pueblo Province* will find some overlap with plant species covered in this book, they will find almost none in the details of their uses.

Finally, we direct you in chapter 12 to a number of other parks and public places that are good travel destinations with features and interpretive information that strongly relate to our story. An annotated checklist of plant species with known uses by past and present native peoples of the Four Corners is incorporated at the end of the book. In this table, species coverage is much more extensive than that for the more common plants described in the main text and includes for each species a thorough summary of the various uses reported in the technical literature.

We have written our book for those who have no formal training in botany or anthropology. Nevertheless, our findings and interpretations are based on material from more than three hundred technical reports and manuscripts, including obscure master's theses, Ph.D. dissertations, and other unpublished papers that are not part of the mainstream reference literature. A selected bibliography is found in the back, and each chapter ends with suggested readings for those who wish to explore a topic in more depth. Additionally, we interviewed many authorities, including Native Americans and academic scholars. We have incorporated as well our own personal observations accrued over a span of many professional years.

In your travels through the Four Corners, you are sure to be impressed by the region's great natural beauty. The geologic wonder of this country is stunning, but when it comes to vegetation and climate, *desert* is the term typically used to describe the vast lower elevations. What does grow sparsely here during most of the year is often prickly, dry, and seldom beckoning. One cannot help but ask the question, How did so many people survive in this now arid, vegetation-poor land for so long? This is the story we tell.

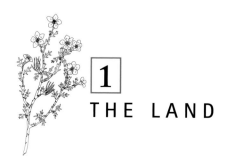

1
THE LAND

HIS IS A LAND of hot summers and frigid winters, meager and unpredictable moisture, relatively sparse vegetation, and rugged, unforgiving landscapes. Such conditions would hardly seem consistent with an environment hospitable to human life, yet this land has been home to humans for at least ten thousand years.

The Four Corners region, extending out from the conjunction of Arizona, New Mexico, Colorado, and Utah, features steep-walled, flat-topped mesas, fractured tablelands, isolated mountain ranges, broad, shallow basins, deep canyons, and very little available water. This majestic landscape is the heart of the Colorado Plateau, a well-defined physiographic province, somewhat larger than the state of Ohio, bordered on the north and east by the Rocky Mountains and Great Plains, on the west by the Wasatch Front and basin-and-range desert country, and at its southwest extremity by the Mogollon Rim.

The Colorado Plateau, actually a series of plateaus, is a geologic uplift feature that was formed early on in our earth's history. It is characterized by sharp-edged landforms and bold

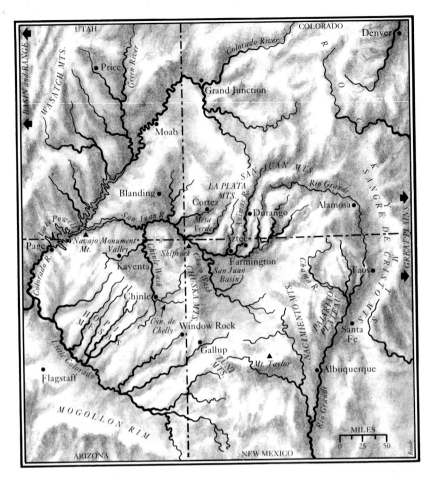

The Colorado Plateau

earth tones. Elevations throughout the province average well over a mile high. The rock one sees in cliffs on the sides of mesas is usually sandstone or limestone; gentler rocky slopes are typically composed of shale, which is softer and more easily eroded.

Outcrops of igneous rock exposed throughout the region attest to volcanic activity that occurred long after the plateau was defined. The most spectacular expression of past volcanism in the Four Corners is Shiprock, a giant black skyscraper that was formed eons ago by molten material squeezed to the surface from great depth. The surrounding soft sediment gradually was eroded, leaving Shiprock, which is today revered by the Navajo as a sacred landform.

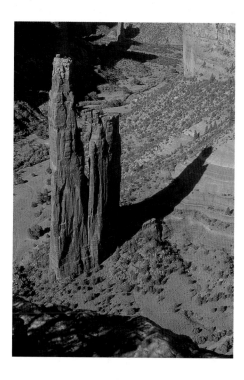

Spider Rock,
an 800-foot sandstone
spire, Canyon de Chelly
National Monument.

At the other geological extreme are the relatively featureless basins found throughout the region, the most prominent being the San Juan Basin with Chaco Canyon at its center. Such basins are the result of accumulated ancient marine sediments and more recently deposited material from surrounding mountain ranges. Where outstanding landforms rise above the basins, such as Fajada Butte in Chaco Canyon, one can easily accept that they were sacred to the ancients. Today, many prominent features are considered inviolate by their descendants.

From its source in the snowcapped San Juan Mountains, the San Juan River cuts across the Colorado Plateau as it descends to the Colorado River, the great runoff receptacle for our region. In fact, the San Juan passes within shouting distance of the tourist monument that heralds the official spot where all four states come together, the absolute Four Corners. Year-round flowing water such as the San Juan provides is scarce in this region. This is arid, semidesert country averaging

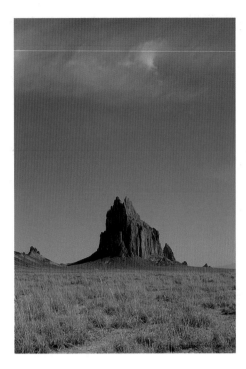

Shiprock,
an expression of past
volcanism, revered by the
Navajo today.

less than ten inches of moisture a year, half of which is delivered by summer thunderstorms, the rest as winter snowfall. Late fall and late spring are the region's driest seasons; sometimes no rainfall moistens the soil for months. Typical average precipitation ranges from barely six inches per year at Monument Valley Navajo Tribal Park to more than eight inches at Chaco Culture National Historical Park and up to eighteen inches at Mesa Verde National Park with its higher elevation. Wet cycles followed by several years of drought, such as occurred during the mid-1990s, are commonplace.

Despite such harsh growing conditions, high diversity of plant and animal life characterizes the region and supported its prehistoric people. Archaic populations were small and mobile enough to move with the rise and fall of sustainable resources. These natural resources were the key to early settlement, although not all locations could support people and few were able to on a sustained basis.

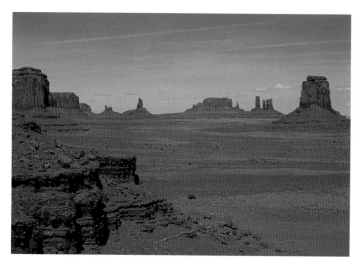

Monument Valley symbolizes Four Corners country.

In the treeless lower valleys and basins, today's visitor typically finds open stands of sagebrush, shadscale, or greasewood shrubs, interspersed with shortgrass vegetation where grazing over the past century has not destroyed it. Above the plains, woodlands comprised of fairly widely spaced piñon pine and juniper trees abound. These woodlands, which define the mesa tops and lower slopes of the islandlike mountain ranges, often support a dense understory of shrubs such as mountain-mahogany or Gambel oak. Higher mountain slopes are forested with ponderosa pines that give way to spruce, fir, and other conifers on the upper reaches of peaks rising above nine thousand feet elevation. Arroyos, those perennially dry, water-carved gullies that seem to define our Southwest, are lined with shrubs, most often rabbitbrush. Ribbons of cottonwood trees delineate the few drainages in which surface water flows or that have a shallow underground water table.

Although much of this area today is rangeland, primarily for cows and sheep, the open country supports abundant wildlife. Besides the ubiquitous cottontails and jackrabbits, small herds of pronghorn antelope graze the shrubby grasslands at lower elevations; deer and occasionally elk inhabit the

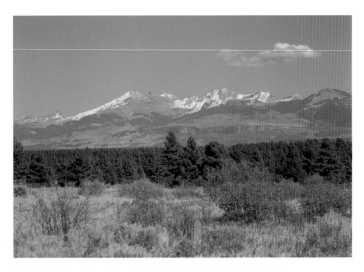

The La Plata Mountains—at over 13,000 feet, the highest landform in the Four Corners region.

mountain ranges and mesa tops. Most of the native mammals— various rodents, raccoons, skunks, and many of the predators— tend to be nocturnal and thus are rarely encountered by the casual observer.

While the region is remarkable for its starkness and arid conditions, much of the Four Corners is too cool and too wet to qualify, technically, as a desert. The true North American subdeserts—the Chihuahuan, Sonoran, and Mojave—lie far to the south and west. The Great Basin Desert covers only portions of the Four Corners. But eleven centuries ago, when our story really begins to unfold, this land had a very different look, as we shall see.

Suggested Reading

Brown, Kenneth A.
1995 *Four Corners: History, Land, and People of the Desert Southwest.* HarperCollins, New York.

Dick-Peddie, William A.
1993 *New Mexico Vegetation: Past, Present and Future.* University of New Mexico Press, Albuquerque.

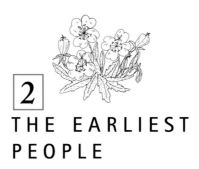

2

THE EARLIEST
PEOPLE

BY THE TIME the first humans are thought to have arrived on the North American continent by way of the Bering Strait land bridge, the last of the hemisphere's great glacial cycles was in recession. Scant but positive evidence collected at ancient campsites indicates that people first occupied the Four Corners area about 9000 B.C., as the climate was warming and the great continental ice sheets were melting. The landscape first inhabited by the early people was thus radically different from that encountered by people today.

Although the geologic landscape was virtually identical to that of modern times, the climate eleven thousand years ago was much wetter and some five to ten degrees Fahrenheit cooler. Water was indeed plentiful. Besides the much more dependable moisture from summer and winter storms, shallow lakes filled some of the low-lying basins, and many streams flowed constantly, carrying runoff from mountain ranges that were far snowier than by current standards.

These cooler, wetter conditions provided for a vastly more lush vegetation, with coniferous forests more widespread and growing at lower elevations than are found today. Spruce, limber pine, and Douglas-fir trees grew at Mesa Verde and in Canyon de Chelly where today more arid piñon-juniper woodlands prevail. The plant community on the mesa tops at Chaco Canyon was dominated by Douglas-fir, Rocky Mountain juniper, limber pine, and, a few centuries later, ponderosa pine, none of which are found now in the shrub-dominated landscape at Chaco. In the lower valleys and basins of the Four Corners region, piñon-juniper woodlands interspersed with expanses of shortgrass savannas and a great deal of sagebrush covered the land.

Even more dramatic was the animal life, most notably the huge mammals that grazed or browsed across the tree-dotted, brushy savannas and the creatures that preyed upon them. Elephantlike mammoths dominated this period, as did other now-extinct fauna such as horses, camels, musk-oxenlike creatures, and giant bison. Great bears, dire wolves, a lion related to the African type, and cougars were the principal meat-eating mammals. In terms of its rich megafauna, before 10,000 B.C. much of the Southwest could be thought of as an extension of the Great Plains, far to the east, and the Great Basin to the northwest. A visit to the Four Corners during the late Pleistocene would have been more akin to taking an African safari than to a tour through modern-day Chaco or Mesa Verde.

We know this mostly from prehistoric animal records. These are relatively easy to track since decay-resistant bones are generally found in shallow ponds where, imbedded in the bottom sediment, they become fossilized. Collections of identifiable bones also turn up in rock shelters or animal-kill processing sites that were used by Paleo-Indians during this period.

Because most plant parts are fragile and become fossilized only under rare conditions, their interpretation is a more difficult proposition. Tree trunks and limbs do withstand the march of time, but it took dendrochronology, the science of tree-ring analysis, to provide solid information about the age and composition of long-gone forests and climatic trends that prevailed. Palynology, the study of fossil pollen, combined with radiocarbon dating has yielded much additional information about what grew in our region long ago. Dendrochronology and palynology also provide information that helps us understand the life and economy of prehistoric peoples. (See chapter 10 for a discussion of Four Corners ethnobotany.)

Perhaps the most fascinating recent approach to understanding bygone environments has been biologists' study of woodrat middens, pioneered by Thomas Van Devender. Woodrats, more commonly called packrats, characteristically collect and store morsels of plant materials, effectively depositing clues to the flora of eras past. Such caches have been discovered in rock crevices, sequestered from the effects of weather and further protected by urine, which acts as a preservative. These crystallized material remains, termed "amberat," can thus be analyzed and identified as to plant species (Betancourt et al. 1990). Over the years, hundreds of middens, or prehistoric dumps, have been examined, and, for any given era, scientists believe that these deposits represent the most accurate picture available of what was growing in a given vicinity at a particular time. Some of the crusted middens represent a veritable herbarium for local flora.

By 9000 B.C., big-game hunters are known to have been living throughout the Great Plains region and likely began to spill over into the Colorado Plateau by this time, if they were not here already, as both regions seem to have supported the same mix of large mammals, especially mammoths and giant bison, that attracted large numbers of roving hunters. Occasional projectile points found mostly along prehistoric lake margins in the Great Basin, well to the northwest of the Four Corners, have been dated to this Paleo-Indian era. Certainly any people living in the region at that time would have depended heavily upon meat for food, although it is assumed that these early mobile hunters also were gatherers of wild plant foods. In our region, however, little direct evidence, such as seed-grinding implements, has been found to confirm that. But elsewhere in North America, and, indeed, throughout the world, animal hunting and plant food gathering were the rule.

The main components of the local diet were to change dramatically over the next two thousand years when most

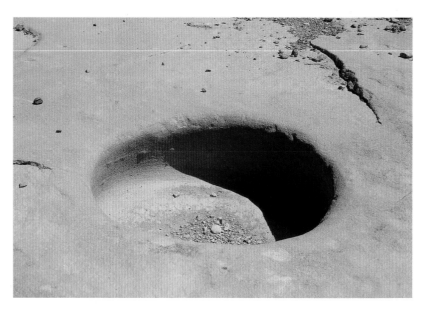

Shallow grinding basins attest to a shift toward a seed diet. Chaco Culture National Historical Park.

megafauna species suffered universal or local extinction. The climate in the greater Southwest was gradually warming, drying up glacier-fed rivers, lakes, and parklands and forcing herds to retreat eastward to the grassy savannas of the Plains. Predation by the increasing numbers of Paleo-Indian hunters also must have taken a toll. Indeed, some researchers believe that Paleo-Indians hastened their own decline with such wasteful hunting practices as driving entire herds over cliffs. By 6000 B.C., most of the megafauna in the Four Corners region had disappeared entirely. Eventually, conditions stabilized and remained so right up to the present, although short- and long-term fluctuations in annual precipitation would regularly occur.

With the onset of more desertlike conditions, new groups of people seem to have moved into our area from further west, heralding what is termed the Archaic Period (5500 B.C. to A.D. 100). Hunting bison and small- to medium-sized game continued to be a way of life. A gradual decline in the number of hunting tools recovered coupled with the appearance and later increase of plant processing devices at archaeologic sites attest to a dietary shift toward more plant foods. Shallow stone basins, or *metates*, for grinding seeds and grains and hand-held grinding stones, or *manos*, regularly surface at sites in the Four Corners. Stone-lined pit ovens that employed heated cobbles for cooking plant foods indicate that the people were becoming less mobile, settling in one location or another for at least brief periods of time before moving on in search of sustenance.

Toward the end of the Archaic Period, many such camp-sites had become quite large. Typically, they were situated near springs, ponds, or other water sources and often in areas that supported a high diversity of wild plants, many of them potential food plants. These early people appear to have developed a pattern of establishing spring and summer camps in sandy locations covered with sagebrush and grass, where grains, weedy annual plants, or sunflower seeds could be harvested, then moving to winter camps in the piñon-juniper zone up on the mesas. Among the wild plant foods known to have been collected for food during the Archaic Period are tansy mustard; fruits of yucca, cactus, and chokecherry; piñon nuts and juniper berries; and seeds of amaranth, goosefoot, purslane, and grass, especially Indian ricegrass.

The invention of weaving—transforming wands of willow, threeleaf sumac, or strips of other wild plants into coiled and twined baskets—allowed for the efficient collection of grass seeds. The charred surfaces of tightly woven baskets from this era suggest that seeds were parched and tossed with hot coals before being stored or processed into meal or gruel.

Other uses of wild plant parts during these times, such as medicinal applications, cannot be proven, but common sense tells us that some unsophisticated form of plant medicine was being practiced long before the record can verify it. One plant that clearly had economic importance during Archaic times was the yucca. Yucca mats, sandals, and other crafted wares designed to make life more comfortable appear in a number of early residence sites. One cave in southeastern Utah that was inhabited off and on for thousands of years throughout the Archaic Period yielded fifty-four sandals. All were fashioned

SUNFLOWER
pg. 258

TANSY MUSTARD
pg. 216

CHOKECHERRY
pg. 139

AMARANTH
pg. 205

PURSLANE
pg. 210

INDIAN RICEGRASS
pg. 194

YUCCA
pg.145

from woven strips of yucca leaves, some with an inner sole padding made from wild grasses.

Gradually, the people left their hunting and gathering practices behind and became food producers and processors. No one knows precisely when the seeds of corn, squash, beans, and bottle gourds made their way northward from central Mexico, where they were cultivated as crops, but by the time of Christ, corn, at least, was being harvested in the American Southwest and added to the wild plants as staples of the human diet. In the place where Arizona, New Mexico, Colorado, and Utah would one day meet, the people had settled in.

Suggested Reading

Betancourt, Julio L., Thomas R. Van Devender and Paul S. Martin
1990 *Packrat Middens—The Last 40,000 Years of Biotic Change*. University of Arizona Press, Tucson.

Cordell, Linda S.
1984 *Prehistory of the Southwest*. Academic Press, San Diego.

Mehringer, Peter J., Jr.
1986 Prehistoric Environments. In *Handbook of North American Indians*, Vol. 11, *Great Basin*, ed. by Warren L. d'Azevedo, pp. 31–50. Smithsonian Institution, Washington, D.C.

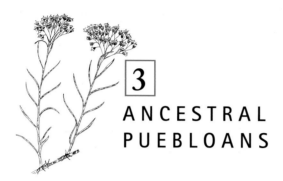

3

ANCESTRAL PUEBLOANS

B Y THE TIME the Ancestral Puebloans,* the people living in the vicinity of the Four Corners, were erecting
permanent architecture, by A.D. 500, they had
acquired the bow and arrow, ceramic production was under
way, and rudimentary farming was becoming a way of life. The
shift to sedentary living correlated with a change in the pattern
of wild-plant food use and, in turn, provided conditions afford-
ing better storage and preservation. With these developments,
a much wider resource base could be tapped.

The civilization of the Ancestral Puebloans represented a
great cultural leap forward from their Archaic forebears. In
fewer than a thousand years, parts of the Four Corners were
counted among the more populated places in North America.
Cities of stone construction featuring "great houses," multistory
buildings with hundreds of rooms and underground ceremonial

---

* The name "Anasazi," popularly applied to these people, the Ancestral Puebloans, is no longer
preferred by modern anthropologists and is rejected by contemporary Puebloans, their direct
descendants. Of Navajo origin, the word has negative connotations. Therefore, throughout
this book we will use the term "Ancestral Puebloans."

chambers (kivas), were built throughout the Four Corners region. Sophisticated agriculture flourished. During this period, A.D. 860–1300, enormous numbers of sites were occupied, not seminomadically, as had been the earlier pattern, but for a generation or longer. And there were spectacular exceptions, such as Chaco Canyon, inhabited for some two and a half centuries.

The incremental progress of this far-reaching culture over a vast region can be examined at national parks at Chaco Canyon, Mesa Verde, and Canyon de Chelly.

Chaco

The term "Chaco Phenomenon" was coined in the 1970s to suggest the uniqueness of a regional system that integrated architectural sites at Chaco Canyon with hundreds of outlying

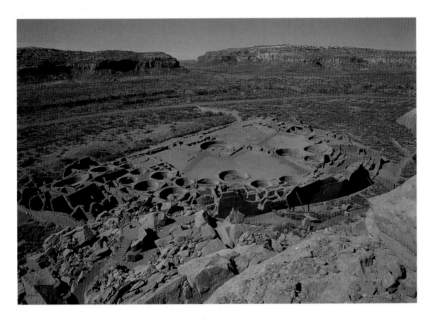

Pueblo Bonito, Chaco Culture National Historical Park

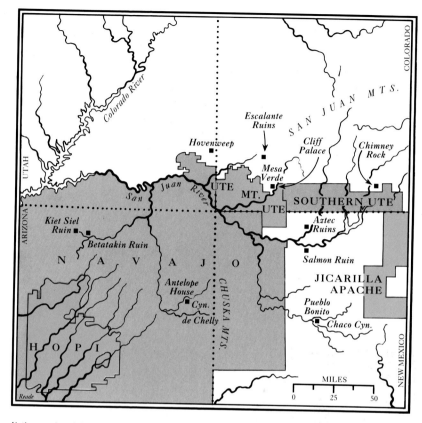

Native peoples of the Four Corners.

districts (outliers) throughout the Four Corners region between about A.D. 900 and 1150. At the center of this vast system were the dozen or so massively scaled buildings and hundreds of smaller unit houses scattered throughout the canyon at Chaco. The famous ruins of Pueblo Bonito, Chetro Ketl, and Peñasco Blanco, three of the largest complexes in the canyon, attest to the remarkable nature of this pre-Puebloan world and give rise to some of its more compelling enigmas. Pueblo Bonito alone comprised some 650 to 800 rooms; the four hundred settlements in and around Chaco have been calculated as capable of housing up to five thousand people; yet the carrying capacity of the land, with its desertic conditions, could not have approached this figure on a year-round basis. This apparent contradiction has led some archaeologists to suggest that Chaco's function was not solely residential but instead included trade and ceremonial uses. Chaco may have been the nexus of a regional food-storage and trade system, served by its immense system of roads.

Alfred V. Kidder, the archaeologist who wrote the first overview of southwestern prehistory, put it this way: ". . . the [Chaco] district is little better than a desert; many parts of it, indeed, are absolutely barren wastes of sand and rock which do not even support the usual dry-country flora of the Southwest. It is almost devoid of springs, has no permanent streams, is subject to severe sandstorms, is blistering hot in summer and bitterly cold in winter. It is hard to see how life in the Chaco could have been anything but a continual struggle for bare existence" (Kidder 1924).

Much of what Kidder reported is as true today as it was a millennium ago. The environment here is not favorable for agriculture. Average annual rainfall is under nine inches, only half of which normally falls during the growing season. The Chacoans had constructed diversion dams across the mouths of side canyons to capture runoff water from the cliffs and used stone-lined canals with headgates to distribute the water to their terraced, gridded gardens. They grew corn, squash, and, to a lesser extent, beans. Despite such advanced water conservation and distribution technology, crop failure must have occurred again and again, forcing the people to rely on stored foodstuffs and to spend more time searching for wild plant foods.

Even in those years when food from the gardens was plentiful, Chacoans continued to depend on wild plant foods, as had their ancestors. The highly nutritious seeds from Indian ricegrass and those of the related dropseed group (*Sporobolus* spp.) were processed in heating pits and turned into mush or bread. Other seeds, such as those of globe-mallow or wild buckwheat, may have been mixed in as ingredients for a soup or stew. Globe-mallow roots were probably used for medicinal purposes, just as they are today by the Hopi. Cactus fruits and

INDIAN RICEGRASS
pg. 194

GLOBE-MALLOW
pg. 231

pads, yucca pods, and, most importantly, piñon nuts were regularly collected to augment the diet of corn and squash. Joint-fir (*Ephedra* spp.) also was collected, but its application was most likely medicinal. The presence of wild tobacco in the plant remains examined at Chaco suggests either smoking or ceremonial use, still the case for many Native Americans. Tobacco (*Nicotiana* spp.), which may have been cultivated at Chaco or acquired by trade, no longer grows wild at Chaco.

PIÑON PINE
pg. 123

JOINT-FIR
pg. 142

Edible weedy annual plants, spring invaders of the garden, constituted another resource. Several of these annual weeds—purslane, with its tart herbage, tansy mustard, amaranth, and goosefoot—paid extra food dividends. "Weedy annuals generally produce a double crop of tender spring greens and abundant tiny seeds in early to late summer," explains ethnobotanist Mollie Toll. "Prolific seed crops and an adaptive advantage under disturbed conditions (such as those surrounding human habitations and fields) encourage human utilization" (Toll 1985). Other weedy plants growing in disturbed sites contributed to the Chacoan diet. Among these were beeplant (probably greens and seeds), blazing star (seeds), and especially the late summer seeds of the prolific native sunflower. Beeplant used to be encouraged as a secondary crop alongside corn by Hopi farmers, and it is possible that centuries earlier Chacoan ancestors also managed beeplant in the same way. Blazing star seeds were being ground into meal by the Hopis as late as the turn of the century. These and other edible seed-producing plants were particularly beneficial, since parched seeds could be stored for use in winter. Most leafy greens would have been eaten immediately; others were hung from the dwelling place ceiling to dry and then stored in bunches, "in which case some of the nutrients would have been lost," Toll attests.

TANSY MUSTARD
pg. 216

AMARANTH
pg. 205

BEEPLANT
pg. 222

BLAZING STAR
pg. 228

In times of famine people will tolerate less desirable foods. Juniper berries and cactus plant parts, such as the desiccated fruits of the prickly pear that adhere to the plants through most of the winter, would have been consumed. During lean times the people probably traveled farther afield to higher, forested ground in their ever-expanding search for piñon nuts, threeleaf sumac berries, netleaf hackberry fruits, and wild game.

JUNIPER
pg. 126

PRICKLY PEAR
pg. 234

THREELEAF
SUMAC
pg. 171

Two of the largest outlier villages in the Chacoan system were Aztec Ruins and Salmon Ruin, located, respectively, alongside the Animas and San Juan rivers due north of Chaco. A visit to either of these sites—both protected and maintained as public parks—makes it obvious that this land is much more amenable to productive farming than was Chaco itself. At Aztec and Salmon, the floodplain soil is richer, annual rainfall is somewhat higher, and the surrounding vegetation is denser and greener, with an apparent higher diversity of plant species. Indeed, at these riverine outliers edible parts from wild riparian plants such as New Mexico olive (fruits), cattails (roots, shoots, and pollen), rushes (seeds), sedges (seeds), and cottonwood (flower parts) must have been part of the diet along with the edible plants more commonly found around Chaco.

COTTONWOOD
pg. 133

There is no good way to estimate the degree of importance of wild game in the Chacoan diet. Available meat sources primarily included cottontail rabbits, jackrabbits, coyotes, and deer. Smaller quantities came from prairie dogs, deer mice, elk, and bighorn sheep, the latter hunted in higher country far from Chaco Canyon itself. While dogs, the sole domesticated mammal, were not an important dietary item, turkeys, which were tamed and penned, provided some food (Gillespie 1993).

The Chacoan road system, a network of hundreds of miles of up to thirty-foot-wide roads leading out from the developed canyon hub, was used for more than trade. Besides the tons of building stone that were quarried annually from the mesas above the great houses at Chaco, vast quantities of wooden beams were used to roof the apartment complexes and ceremonial kivas. More than fifty thousand timbers are estimated to have gone into the construction of Pueblo Bonito alone. While the earliest builders at Chaco must have depended upon nearby sources for timbers, mainly cottonwood, piñon pine, and some ponderosa pine, the supply of local wood was soon depleted, and tree harvests expanded outward, finally reaching the surrounding mountains. Thus, a major function of the road system was for hauling logs (Windes and Ford 1996).

Some of the woods regularly utilized in Chaco home construction did not grow on the nearby mesas. Douglas-fir was a frequent beam element, and the best source for it was the Chuska Mountains, fifty miles to the west of Chaco. But we know Chacoans traveled much farther than that. They could have brought in spruce from Mount Taylor, about sixty-five miles to the south, but white fir, another timber used in Chaco construction, occurs neither in the Chuskas nor on Mount Taylor. For this wood, Chacoans would have trekked to the Nacimiento Mountains, eighty miles to the east, or to the La Platas, even further to the north. It is estimated that the collection and transportation of timbers accounted for about one-third of the total effort in each construction project and that it was an activity that went on every year (Vivian 1990).

Chacoans had neither wheeled vehicles nor draft animals. The absence of transportation scars indicates that the logs were carried rather than dragged or rolled. The image we have is of work forces made up of many people with logs shouldered, marching along the roads leading to the canyon. Of course, members of outlying communities such as Aztec might have provided some of the timber and labor as part of their contribution to the Chacoan system.

As noted, the harvesting of trees for construction thinned the local woodlands that had been comprised of piñon and juniper trees as well as some ponderosa pine. Piñon and juniper may have been important sources of fuel in the earliest days, but when these trees became scarce, the land was scoured for mature greasewood, sagebrush, and fourwing saltbush, all of which burn with a hot flame. Construction also took a toll on plants growing at the bottom of Chaco Wash, such as cottonwood, common reed (*Phragmites communis*), and bulrush (*Scirpus* spp.), the last of which also was a food-producing group of plants. Reed and bulrush were used in roof thatching but are gone from the canyon today. Yuccas were another heavily utilized group of plants. Although they are no longer common in the vicinity of Chaco, they were a prehistoric mainstay for making cordage, mats, and a host of other items.

COMMON REED
pg. 197

Deforestation, depletion of other useful wild plants, and the shift in dietary meat from deer to rabbits and small rodents, a sequence evident from archaeological excavations, were all symptomatic of the severe stress wrought upon the environment by its human population. Whereas most of us living in the industrial world today recognize environmental warning signals, Chacoans may only have been puzzled by what was happening in their natural world.

Other less obvious problems were mounting. Many centuries of continuous irrigation had probably led to excessive accumulation of salts in the soil. Erosion over a denuded landscape would have diminished its usability and lowered irrigation-system channels below the level of the fields, making further irrigation at that site impossible without building new canals. To top if off, a cycle of unusually dry weather lasting nearly sixty years set in about the twelfth century, causing regional water tables to drop even more. Depleted resources and failed crops soon translated into disintegration of the Chacoan culture; unknown cultural or religious factors also may have played a role. By A.D. 1120 construction using new wood had ended at Chaco, and by A.D. 1150, the Chaco Phenomenon was about over, its population dispersed to the regions lying at the periphery. Drought certainly was a factor, but "the Anasazis themselves also inflicted fatal blows to the fragile desert environment" (Diamond 1986).

Mesa Verde

Where did the people of Chaco go? Survivors are believed to have drifted in all directions, moving into the upland area surrounding the San Juan Basin. They may have migrated westward into the Chuska Mountains or even farther west into the region that was soon to become the homeland for the Hopi, who today occupy the mesas and washes north and east of Flagstaff. Some of those who went south probably settled in the Zuni Mountains or traveled farther east to the flanks of the Jemez and Sandia mountains. Others possibly moved northward, becoming integrated with their ethnic relatives who had

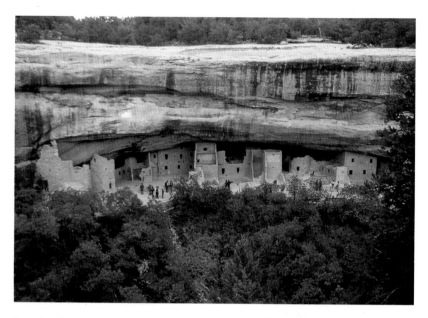

Spruce Tree House, Mesa Verde National Park.

long been living on the green tableland of Mesa Verde and at numerous other sites in present-day southwestern Colorado and southeastern Utah. Whether or not Chacoans were part of their number, by the thirteenth century the people of Mesa Verde had come into their own, many of them living in those spectacular dwellings for which the present-day national park is justly famed.

The physical environment at Mesa Verde contrasts sharply with the landscape we have been describing for Chaco. More than a thousand feet higher in elevation and much closer to the flanks of the southern Rocky Mountains, annual precipitation at Mesa Verde is double that of Chaco Canyon. Instead of semi-desert vegetation, the Mesa Verde tablelands harbor a dense piñon-juniper woodland, with Douglas-fir growing on the north-facing slopes and in some of the sheltered canyons. One also finds here a much higher diversity of plant life within a day's reach of the mesa tops.

Farming was the main livelihood for the Ancestral

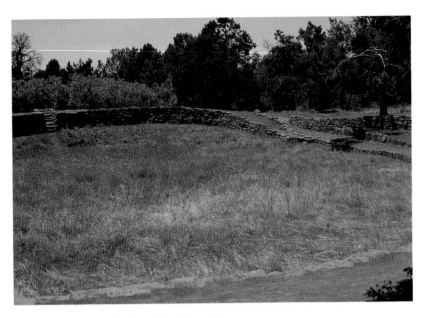

Mummy Lake, Mesa Verde National Park.

Puebloans living here, just as it was at Chaco. While most years were wet enough to permit dryland farming of corn and other crops, the presence of prehistoric reservoirs, ditches, and check dams indicates the practice of water conservation here, too. Most of these devices at Mesa Verde exist on a smaller scale, suggesting that many of them were the work of individual households, although one huge walled-in depression now known as Mummy Lake appears to have been a reservoir, probably requiring a community effort to construct and operate. The more than one thousand rough sandstone-block dams that have been recorded from Mesa Verde drainages are notable in that at least part of their purpose seems to have been to accumulate terraces of silt behind them, ideal places for planting crops. Small, seasonally occupied stone-block quarters often were built in the ravines that contained these dams and terraces, further indicating that planting and harvesting were often done on a family-by-family basis.

Whereas Mesa Verdeans ate more corn than any other plant food, two other cultigens, squash and, to a lesser extent, beans, were mainstays of their diet. They also relied heavily on wild plants that thrived in disturbed soil and grew in and around their garden plots and may well have been manipulated, or at least encouraged, by the farmers. "Disturbed soil" plants such as Rocky Mountain beeplant greens and seedpods, groundcherry pods, as well as amaranth, goosefoot, and wild purslane seeds contributed to the nutritional mix. A host of other plant parts that could have been collected from the mesa tops and canyon bottoms, such as prickly pear seeds and pads, fourwing saltbush fruits, and piñon pine nuts, would have rounded out the diet in any given year.

ROCKY MOUNTAIN
BEEPLANT
pg. 222

FOURWING
SALTBUSH
pg. 152

We know this from information yielded by dozens of coprolites, or desiccated feces, of prehistoric residents of Mesa Verde country that have been collected on-site and analyzed in the laboratory (see chapter 10). Archaeologists once interpreted prehistoric subsistence patterns based on easy-to-examine plant remains recovered from excavations. Now they recognize and use the scientific data that coprolites contain; indeed, this information greatly increases our understanding of the role wild plants played in the diets of early people.

Capitalizing on Mesa Verde's greater plant diversity, the people also collected a number of plants not found or at least not common at Chaco. Added to the Ancestral Puebloan menu at Mesa Verde were Gambel oak acorns, buffaloberry (*Shepherdia* spp.) and chokecherry fruits, and peppergrass seeds.

GAMBEL OAK
pg. 136

CHOKECHERRY
pg. 139

PEPPERGRASS
pg. 219

Marilyn Colyer, natural resource manager for Mesa Verde, speculates that many more species of wild plants known to be dietary items for native peoples living in other places in the Southwest during historic times must also have been used by the Ancestral Puebloans at Mesa Verde, even though their remains have yet to be detected in coprolites. Among such potential foods are the swollen root nodes of chickweed (*Stellaria* spp.), fruits of snowberry and Utah serviceberry and the bulbous roots of biscuit-root (*Lomatium* spp.), wild onion, and wild sego lily (*Calochortus* spp.). Other edible plants that

SNOWBERRY
pg. 183

UTAH
SERVICEBERRY
pg. 159

SEGO LILY
pg. 199

are common at Mesa Verde today, and thus good candidates for use by the people who once lived there, include evening primrose (roots of young plants, cooked), mulesears (*Wyethia arizonica*; cooked roots), arrowleaf balsamroot (*Balsamorhiza sagittata*; young shoots, leaves and roots), and Oregon grape (*Berberis repens*; berries).

MULESEARS
pg. 261

ARROWLEAF
BALSAMROOT
pg. 261

OREGON GRAPE
pg. 155

Like all prehistoric societies, Mesa Verdeans experienced times of food surplus and times of scarcity. Compared with Chaco, here there would have been a greater variety of marginal food plants to draw upon during periods of famine. The mucilaginous inner bark of many trees contains nutrients and is edible, if not tasty. In lean times, Navajo and Ute Indians are known to have harvested the inner bark of piñon pine and juniper trees, and it seems probable that the Ancestral Puebloans of Mesa Verde would have done so as well, since these conifers occur everywhere on the mesa. Another item consumed during famines is the berry of the ubiquitous juniper tree. In the past century, Pueblo Indians living south of Mesa Verde have gathered this dry, resinous fruit as a last resort. The

UTAH JUNIPER
pg. 126

principal juniper species at Mesa Verde is Utah juniper (*Juniperus osteosperma*), and it has much larger berries than one-seed juniper (*J. monosperma*), which grows in the modern Pueblo Province. Thus, juniper's inner bark and berries could have been important food items when other foods were scarce.

When it comes to seeds, pollen, or other parts of herbaceous plants, we have no way of knowing which wild plants were ingested as food and which were used for medicine (See chapter 9). Woody plant remains, however, often can be easily tied to specific uses, such as ancient crafts, tools, implements, or ceremonial objects. At Mesa Verde, hoes made from Gambel oak, serviceberry, and mountain-mahogany have been found among the ruins. Wooden dishes were crafted from softer wood, often Douglas-fir or pine. When the bow and arrow was invented or introduced to the region from the outside after A.D. 400, the bow typically was made of oak, willow, or cottonwood, the arrows of willow or common reed, and the arrow points often were carved from cliff fendlerbush stems.

MOUNTAIN-
MAHOGANY
pg. 165

Baskets were woven from split willow wands, threeleaf sumac, or rabbitbrush. When pottery was introduced after A.D. 500, it was often decorated with black paint produced from the iron-rich shoots of beeplant or tansy mustard. Piñon pine pitch was used to waterproof the baskets and to glue other things together.

WILLOW
pg. 130

RABBITBRUSH
pg. 188

Fibers from banana yucca plants, which today grow everywhere on the mesas, were converted into cordage and various textiles. Wider strips were woven into mats, sandals, tump straps, and headbands. The spine-tipped leaf ends of banana yucca still connected to fiber made excellent needles and thread, and the tips alone were used to make hairbrushes.

BANANA YUCCA
pg. 145

During most of the time that Mesa Verde was populated by Ancestral Puebloans, from A.D. 500 until 1300, the people lived on top of the mesas. It was not until about A.D. 1200 that the cliff alcoves were occupied in large numbers and the famous cliff houses were created. The reasons why so many of the great structures were built in such hard-to-reach places are unknown, but defensive positioning, protection from the elements, or religious practices may all have had a role in the development of these dwellings.

If Frijoles Canyon at Bandelier National Monument was the most beautiful setting for habitation during this period, then the cliffs of Mesa Verde National Park are surely the most spectacular. Yet these well-preserved dwellings were minor settlements and really an aberration compared to the much larger communities in the nearby fertile farmland of the Montezuma Valley to the north and west of Mesa Verde and to the canyon and mesa communities that extended far to the southwest. Altogether within the Four Corners region more than 100,000 sites of this era have been mapped, and some archaeologists have estimated that three times that number await discovery. While this region has one of the highest concentrations of prehistoric sites in the world, only a few were occupied at any one time.

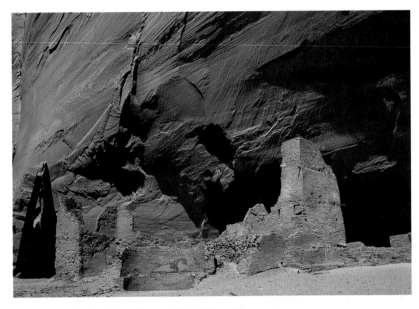

Antelope House, Canyon de Chelly National Monument.

Canyon de Chelly

The excavation of Antelope House in Canyon de Chelly National Monument, Arizona, by the National Park Service in the 1970s provided some of the best information relating to wild plant uses by Ancestral Puebloans. At least seventy-eight species of plants known to have been used for food at one time or another throughout the Southwest were recovered in refuse heaps found in this eighty-nine-room structure, which was small by the standards of many other sites. Three times as many more edible species grew within a short distance of the eight-hundred-year-old pueblo. The analysis of coprolites reveals that the diet remained relatively unchanged over a long period of time and that no major pathological organisms infected the people.

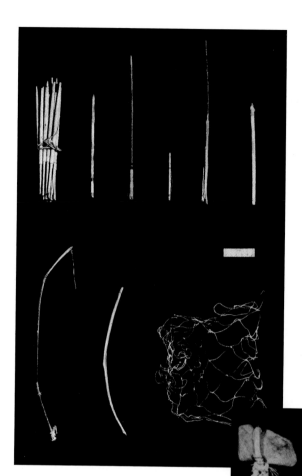

TOP
Hunting equipment from Antelope House (clockwise
from top left): bundle of mountain-mahogany arrow
points; arrows made from common reed, greasewood, and groundsel; net of yucca fiber; bows of
Gambel oak and willow.

RIGHT
Stone axes hafted with Gambel oak from Antelope
House, Canyon de Chelly.

In addition to food remains, hundreds of wooden and other plant-material artifacts were recovered, indicating the use of more than a dozen different kinds of native trees and shrubs. One of the most fascinating discoveries was the more than one hundred little bundles of wild plants, most of them bound with strips of yucca, threeleaf sumac, or willow. Many of the bundles contain sprigs of various wild plants that have known medicinal uses; these might have been the Ancestral Puebloan healers' tools, or perhaps they were part of an ordinary family's medicine cabinet. Other bundles contained raw materials— willow, common reed, cattails, sumac—that could have been collected and stored for craft or other special projects.

The investigation of woven material at Antelope House proves that the people grew cotton, suggests that this was a textile manufacturing area, and reveals that weaving was usually done in kivas. Recovered woven objects ranged from yarns and tapestries to covers for baby cradles. Counterparts of nearly all the tools the Hopi Indians used in historic times for ginning, spinning, weaving, and sewing were found at Antelope House, one more positive indication of the link between the people of this era and contemporary Puebloans.

The communities at Mesa Verde, Canyon de Chelly, and most of the Ancestral Puebloan sites on much of the Colorado Plateau were abandoned by A.D. 1300 or shortly thereafter. The last quarter of the thirteenth century was marked by drought and crop failures. It appears that many of the environmental stress problems that had occurred at Chaco and probably had driven the people out of that canyon, occurred again less than one hundred years later in these new settings. As at Chaco, religious or other cultural factors may have been partly responsible for the people's departure, but the main impetus appears to lie in the fact that the growing population's needs in the thirteenth century exceeded the local environment's production capacity.

The Ancestral Puebloans fanned out to the west, south, and east to new locations where water was available throughout the year. They went to places such as the Little Colorado River north of present-day Flagstaff, the Chama Valley in northern

New Mexico, the Pajarito Plateau west of Santa Fe, and the Rio Grande corridor, where settlement already had begun centuries before but where much vacant land remained. "Perhaps new lands and dynamic new communities in the south provided a 'pull' on northern San Juan populations that reinforced whatever 'push' was being exerted by environmental or other problems in their homeland" (Van West 1993).

The story of this people's settlement along the Rio Grande drainage, how they became the forerunners to the inhabitants of New Mexico's nineteen contemporary pueblos, and how they continued to incorporate wild plants into many aspects of their lives is a volume unto itself (see *Wild Plants of the Pueblo Province*, Dunmire and Tierney, 1995).

In the next chapter we turn our attention to the Hopi of northeastern Arizona. Possibly more than any other modern people, the Hopi can link their heritage directly to the people of Mesa Verde, Hovenweep, Canyon de Chelly, and to the myriad prehistoric villages that once thrived in the Four Corners region. The Hopi's own word for ancestors who occupied these sites is *Hisatsinon*, which translates to "people of long ago."

Suggested Reading

Brody, J.J.
1990 *The Anasazi: Ancient Indian People of the American Southwest.* Rizzoli, New York.

Cordell, Linda S.
1984 *Prehistory of the Southwest.* Academic Press, San Diego.

Dunmire, William W. and Gail D. Tierney
1995 *Wild Plants of the Pueblo Province: Exploring Ancient and Enduring Uses.* Museum of New Mexico Press, Santa Fe.

Lekson, Stephen H., Rena Swentzell and Catherine M. Cameron
1993 *Ancient Land, Ancestral Places: Paul Logsdon in the Pueblo Southwest.* Museum of New Mexico Press, Santa Fe.

Morris, Don P., ed.
1986 *Archaeological Investigations at Antelope House.* National
Park Service, Washington, D.C.

Vivian, R. Gwinn
1990 *The Chacoan Prehistory of the San Juan Basin.* Academic
Press, San Diego.

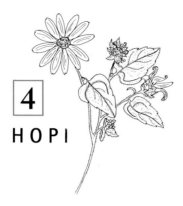

4
HOPI

I T WOULD BE A MISTAKE to think of Hopi country as having been populated solely by people who had migrated from the northern prehistoric pueblos. Old Oraibi, a village on Hopi Third Mesa, had been inhabited for at least a hundred years before the great Ancestral Puebloan pullout about A.D. 1300. In fact, Old Oraibi is the oldest continuously inhabited town in the United States. Unlike most of the other tribes of Indians who moved into the Four Corners arena in the post-Chacoan period—the Utes, Paiutes, Navajo, and Apache—the Hopi were there first and there they remained.

The Hopi are among the most conservative native peoples in the Southwest. For the most part, they have maintained their time-honored ways of life. Lacking a written language, their oral traditions and the perpetuation of their conventional ways have supplied the information that has enabled anthropologists to bridge the gap of time and make educated guesses as to how their ancestors, the previously discussed Ancestral Puebloans, interacted with the world around them.

Like their ancestors, Hopi people are farmers first and foremost. The tradition of farming, principally corn but also squash, beans, gourds, and cotton, was certainly carried over from prehistoric times. The Spanish later introduced other cultivated plants, including lima beans, chile peppers, domestic onions, watermelons, and especially peach trees.

Today's visitors to the austere landscape of the three Hopi mesas might well marvel that these ancestral refugees from the north chose to settle here. That they could have survived as farmers is even more intriguing, given a harsh environment where rainfall averages less than eight inches a year, barely enough for growing corn without irrigation. The answer is that the mesas are underlain by shallow layers of sandstone below which are sheets of shale and clay that are impervious to water penetration. Water trapped in the sandstone during wet years is released slowly to the surface in the form of springs at the mesa edges, providing a reliable source of domestic water.

Over the millennia, windblown sand has accumulated in the valleys between these mesas. The sand absorbs moisture from unpredictable, often violent storms and acts as a subterranean reservoir. Deep-rooted crops are planted over these sandy aquifers or in runoff zones where summer thunderstorm water spreads out at the mouths of the arroyos descending from the mesas. Like the Chacoans and Mesa Verdeans before them, the Hopi built stone dams across the arroyos to slow and spread water from the deluges. And like those ancestors, they tried (and many still do) to have at least a year's supply of corn safely stored as insurance against the inevitable years of crop failure.

Most varieties of corn are altogether unsuitable for the planting depth (eight to sixteen inches) that is required to prevent early desiccation. Specialized strains were required that had developed a greatly elongated growth form capable of reaching the surface. Additionally, such strains would have to develop a single long taproot that could deeply penetrate the sand and capture the available moisture. These strains, today known as Hopi corn, typically produce hard and brightly colored, sometimes multicolored kernels. The yield from each plant is surprisingly high. To the untrained eye, the growth form of this corn appears to be stunted, but in this region of ferocious desiccating winds a compact form is advantageous.

Hopi corn is the product of a long line of evolution and travel. Starting with the first tiny-kerneled corn that was domesticated in the highlands of Mexico more than five thousand years ago, the spread of a more advanced, larger variety into the Southwest began some two thousand years later. Varieties that were grown at Chaco and afterward throughout the Four Corners region finally made their way south again. No wonder that corn is so revered and honored by these people.

The Hopi have always been tolerant of and encouraged the growth of useful wild plants that volunteer into their garden plots. Bee-balm (*Monarda menthaefolia*), wild tobacco (*Nicotiana* spp.), wild potato, and beeplant have recently been among their semicultivated wild plants. Weedy annuals such as amaranth and wild dock (*Rumex hymenosepalus*), which can offer nutritious leafy greens to the cook pot in early spring, used to be left unmolested in the otherwise carefully tended fields. Even today some traditional Hopi farmers encourage and harvest such wild plants found growing alongside their corn or beans.

AMARANTH
pg. 205

As will be apparent in the descriptions of useful wild plants that begins on page 123 and in the annotated list of useful

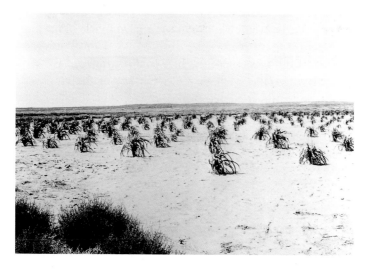

Hopi cornfield, 1935

plants found in the back, the Hopi have maintained an enduring tradition of seeking out and harvesting from the wild yucca fruits, spring greens, nuts, seeds, and cactus fruits. Thus, although Hopi people are predominantly farmers, they continue to be gatherers as well.

In addition to the more than one hundred species that have been collected over the years for food and medicine, many other species were and still are the main ingredients for preparing pigment solutions used to dye wool used in blankets, cotton used in clothing, and materials used in woven baskets (Colton 1965). Plant parts were once routinely employed to make hunting and farming tools and items for everyday use. At least eight different plants are incorporated in the crafting of the flutes and rhythm instruments that are so much a part of Hopi religious ceremonies.

The Hopi were probably the earliest people of the Southwest whose use of wild plants attracted academic attention. In the 1890s, archaeologist J. Walter Fewkes took a brief detour from his ongoing studies of Indian ruins and ceremonies to focus on Hopi use of plants. "I believe they have employed for food as large a number of plants as any aborigines of America," he explained, "and that they have more than once bridged over the failure of the staple crop, maize, by other plant foods" (Fewkes 1896). His 1896 article in the journal *American Anthropologist*, entitled "A Contribution to Ethnobotany," was one of the first published uses of the term "ethnobotany." But our best understanding of the Hopi wild plant connection is largely a dividend from the studies Alfred E. Whiting made in the 1930s. His subsequent treatise, *Ethnobotany of the Hopi* (Whiting 1939), is one of the most comprehensive for any native group living in North America.

Suggested Reading

Brew, J. O.
1979   Hopi Prehistory and History to 1850. In *Handbook of North American Indians*, Vol. 9, *Southwest*, ed. by Alfonso Ortiz, pp. 514–23. Smithsonian Institution, Washington, D.C.

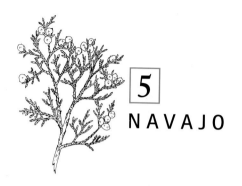

5

NAVAJO

THE PREVAILING VIEW among archaeologists and anthropologists is that the Navajo, along with the Apache, are descendants of people who originally entered North America from Asia via the second major migration across the Bering Strait land bridge. This migration is thought to have occurred sometime between twelve and fourteen thousand years ago. Following their entry into the New World, these hunters, foragers, and fishermen are believed to have roamed the northern forests and plains of Canada and Alaska for many thousands of years. One of the linguistic divisions of these people, the Athapaskans, appears to have been the ancestors of modern Navajos and Apaches; another group were the predecessors of the Ute and Paiute Indians. The name Navajo is a Spanish corruption of a Tewa-Pueblo language term that means "great planted fields." Contemporary Navajos call themselves Diné, "the people."

It was not until shortly before Coronado and his Spanish followers invaded the Rio Grande corridor from Mexico in 1540 that the Navajo line of Athapaskans moved into north-

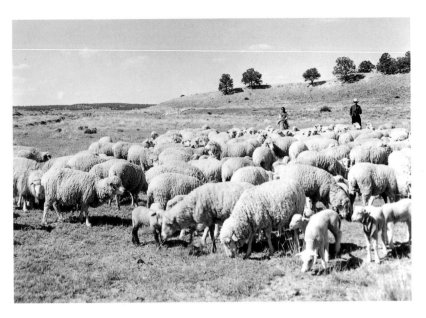

Sheep grazing on Navajoland, 1930s.

eastern New Mexico from the north. In time they slowly migrated westward, occupying the open, semidesert mesa-and-range country at lower elevations in the Four Corners region. They did not enter Canyon de Chelly in Arizona, one of their revered places today, until the last half of the eighteenth century.

When they first arrived in the Southwest, the Navajo are thought to have been nomadic hunters, wild plant gatherers, and, at times, raiders. After they crossed paths with the Spaniards, however, their life-style changed dramatically.

Among the livestock that the Spanish introduced into the Rio Grande corridor at the end of the sixteenth century were sheep. It didn't take long before the Navajo acquired some of these animals that were so admirably suited to browsing the low, dry shrubs that dot the Four Corners landscape. Eventually, the Navajo embraced a pastoral life centered around their roving bands of sheep, and by the beginning of the twentieth century, the tribe owned one million of these cloven-hoofed animals. "Moving seasonally with their flocks, they developed a way of life so closely tied to the land that they came to regard themselves not as immigrants from the north but as natives who emerged from right up out of the ground itself. The vast deserts and canyons of the Four Corners region became a holy land" (Brown 1995).

Although by tradition these people had not been agriculturists, they probably learned how to plant corn, squash, and beans from the Puebloans and were definitely growing corn at the time of the Spanish *Entrada* in 1540. In time they became first-class farmers, which they still are today.

More species of wild plants—some 450 species—are associated with Navajo medicine than with any other type of use. Every known disease or ailment and every approach to better health has one or more plants associated with it as a cure or benefit. Some plants have dozens of medicinal applications. Navajo culture allows many herbal medicines to be used by ordinary citizens without an accompanying ceremonial rite or the supervision of a tribal medicine man or woman. Tradition

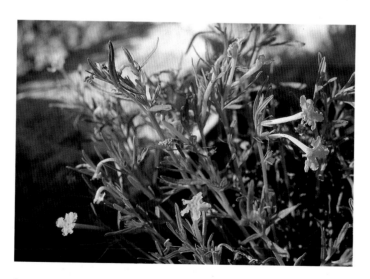

Puccoon, a Navajo medicine plant.

does require that a prayer be offered whenever plants are collected in the wild for whatever purpose.

Navajo "Life Medicine" is a mixture of parts from several different plants that are known to have special healing powers. An extraordinary number of plant species may be used to concoct the various Life Medicine mixtures, although a few, including sagebrush (*Artemisia* spp.), puccoon (*Lithospermum multiflorum*), and the wild buckwheats (*Eriogonum* spp.), seem to top the list.

SAGEBRUSH pg. 191

WILD BUCKWHEAT pg. 202

Of course, some herbal medicine treatments do require a ceremony conducted under the direction of a medicine man. Devotees of Tony Hillerman mysteries are familiar with the Blessingway, the central ceremony in Navajo religion that serves to maintain harmony and balance for the people. This and other rituals incorporate pollen or other plant parts in the ceremonial practice. Chants often are accompanied by the administration of lotions, infusions, or other preparations brewed from special plants. Prior to several ceremonies, participants are required to cleanse themselves by drinking a strong concoction made up of a variety of wild herbs that act as an emetic, or they may prepare for the ceremony by bathing in frothy wild yucca-root suds. As some sacred or ritual uses of plants are not meant to be shared with outsiders, we have not revealed any such use that isn't already widely known.

The availability of sheep and goats provided a dependable food supply that allowed the Navajo population to expand. As sheep tending became a way of life, it was not long before they began to shear the wool and weave the spun fleece from their animals. Pueblo Indians had introduced the Navajo to the upright loom, and by about A.D. 1650 Navajo women had learned the art of weaving. Interestingly, in Pueblo cultures, including the Hopi, it was the men who were weavers, whereas among the Navajo, only women are weavers.

By the mid-1800s Navajo women were producing rugs for wholesale. Eventually, these women had far-outstripped Puebloans and most other cultures' ability to create highly varied and extraordinarily patterned rugs and blankets for which they are so famous today. The connection between wild plants

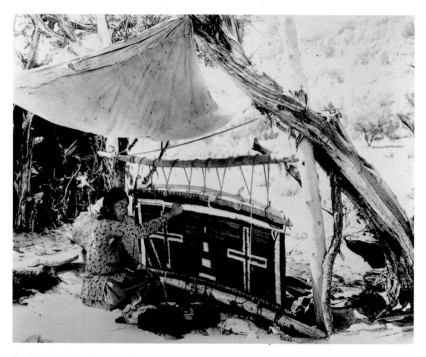

Navajo woman weaving on traditional loom, undated.

and Navajo weaving is overwhelming. Wool is cleaned in a bath made of crushed yucca roots and water. Looms were fabricated from several native woods. Some rugs had extraneous plant or animal material intentionally woven into them. More than three dozen wild plant species were used for dyes, which were fixed with a mordant made from boiled juniper ashes (Bryan and Young 1940). Recent experimentation by Navajo weavers has greatly expanded the list of native plants that may be used to create dyes.

Navajo people always have lived close to the land, and they maintain a huge store of knowledge about wild plants and continue to apply this knowledge to nearly every aspect of their lives. Some 240 species of wild plants were once used by the Kayenta, a single group of Navajo who live in the region of Canyon de Chelly and Monument Valley (Wyman and Harris

1951). The number expands greatly when the Navajo Nation as a whole is considered.

The importance of the connection between wild plant use and Navajo people has been recognized and fostered by modern Navajo educators. At Chinle, Arizona, just west of Canyon de Chelly National Monument, the school district has developed a "Plants of Navajoland" teaching unit within the science curriculum. The aim is to promote student awareness of wild plants and to instill a respect for the natural environment. First published in 1995, this curriculum includes full-color student and teacher manuals in both Navajo and English. The manuals cover the identification and traditional Navajo uses of dozens of local plant species. The introduction includes the following observation by curriculum center coordinator Gloria Grant Means. "We are aware that what we have produced is revolutionary. Revolutionary in the sense that we went back to learn some of the traditional teaching and methods used by our ancestors to observe, respect and share the knowledge of what was given to us through nature."

It is in the nature of Navajo people to approach wild plant collection with conservation in mind. Plants are picked only as needed, limited to the amount necessary. If one species is being collected for healing or medicinal purposes, it is common for a prayer and sometimes an offering to be presented to a nearby plant of the same species. The healthiest specimens are left to perpetuate the species.

In her marvelously poetic book, *Pieces of White Shell: A Journey to Navajoland*, Terry Tempest Williams sums up the Navajo-wild plant connection: "Plants yield their secrets to those who know them. They can weep the colors of chokecherry tears, purplish-brown, into a weaver's hands. They can be backbones for baskets holding the blessings of *Kinaaldá* [a Blessingway ceremony]. Cedar bark and sage can purify; Indian paintbrush soothes an ailing stomach. Juniper ash water creates blue cornmeal. Petals of larkspur are sprinkled in ceremony. Native plants are a repository. They hold our health. A Navajo medicine man relies on plants as we rely on pharmacies" (Williams 1983).

Today with tribal membership approaching a quarter-million people, Navajo are the most populous of all Native Americans living in the United States, and the Navajo Nation exerts a powerful influence on life throughout the Four Corners region. The Navajo Reservation in northwestern New Mexico, northeastern Arizona, and southeastern Utah is by far the largest of all Indian reservations, about equal in size to the states of New Hampshire, Vermont, and Massachusetts combined. It covers some twenty-five thousand square miles of arid canyon, mesa, and plateau country and encompasses several forested mountain ranges.

Monument Valley in northeast Arizona and spilling into Utah is probably the best-known natural landscape of Navajoland. Established as a tribal park in 1958 and drawing some half-million visitors yearly, its spellbinding scenery exemplifies the fantastic geology of the Four Corners. A plethora of trading posts, gift shops featuring Navajo-made crafts, and small museums is scattered across the reservation, many in out-of-the-way places.

Suggested Reading

Kent, Kate Peck
1985 *Navajo Weaving: Three Centuries of Change.* School of American Research, Santa Fe.

Mayes, Vernon O. and Barbara Bayless Lacy
1989 *Nanisé : A Navajo Herbal.* Navajo Community College Press, Tsaile, AZ.

Williams, Terry Tempest
1983 *Pieces of White Shell: A Journey to Navajoland.* University of New Mexico Press, Albuquerque.

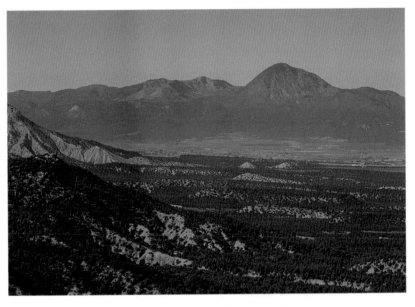

The Sleeping Ute, revered landmark of the Ute Mountain Ute
Indian Reservation.

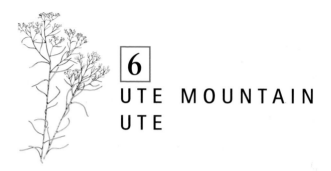

6
UTE MOUNTAIN UTE

RCHAEOLOGISTS and anthropologists seem to agree that Ute Indians have occupied a large area of the northwestern Four Corners region for at least five hundred years, longer than any other modern tribe living in this area.

Where these people came from is still debated. One school maintains that the Utes migrated from western Canada and even Alaska, another that they moved in from the deserts of southern Nevada and southeastern California. Still others cite the continuity in material culture and life-styles between Archaic period Indians who once occupied the Four Corners and the Ute, suggesting that Ute Indians may have occupied portions of the Colorado Plateau for many thousands of years. The dilemma is that few sites attributed to prehistoric Ute occupation have been discovered, and that most research has been directed toward Ancestral Puebloan and Archaic cultures.

By the time the Ute Indians migrated into the area north of the Four Corners around A.D. 1300, Ancestral Puebloans had already abandoned their numerous Four Corners sites, including Aztec, Mesa Verde, Hovenweep, and Canyon de Chelly, and settled along the Rio Grande and points west. Territory that was newly occupied by the Ute soon was surrounded by other recently arrived Indian tribes. Arapaho, Cheyenne, Kiowa, Comanche, and Sioux claimed the lands to the north and east, while Shoshone, Snake Indians, and Paiute dominated land to the west. Athapaskan-speaking Navajo and Apache blocked the way south of the Four Corners. The Ute themselves were most closely related to the Paiute and Shoshone, all speaking the same language.

It was not long before Utes living west of the Four Corners broke up into half a dozen or so bands. One of these, the Weeminuche, eventually occupied southwestern Colorado and became known as the Ute Mountain Ute, so named after the beautiful, nearly 10,000-foot-high mountain, now affectionately called "The Sleeping Ute," that rises to the west of their headquarters at Towaoc, Colorado.

Before the acquisition of Spanish horses and the increased mobility and range they afforded, Ute Mountain Ute subsisted on hunting deer, elk, and antelope, and capturing many kinds of smaller animals. A significant part of their diet was supplied by plants. Seeds, such as those of yellow beeplant (*Cleome lutea*) and various grasses; piñon pine nuts; vitamin-rich berries from native plants such as silvery buffaloberry (*Shepherdia argentea*), chokecherry, and Utah juniper; and roots from a number of wild plants were mainstays. The inner bark from aspen trees growing on the mountains to the north was considered a great delicacy. They supplemented with snakes, lizards, and creatures of the insect world such as grasshoppers, caterpillars, and eggs of various insects.

YELLOW BEEPLANT
pg. 222

ASPEN
pg. 133

The colonizers from Spain living along the Rio Grande had no intention of allowing Indians living within Spanish territory to gain possession of horses; their own complex rules forbade Indians even from riding horses. But great numbers of horses were abandoned when the Spanish were temporarily forced out of New Mexico by the Pueblo Indian Revolt of 1680, and by their reconquest in 1692–3 the question of mobility among tribes in the area had changed irrevocably. The Ute

Indians became the first western Indians to own horses in great numbers. They could now hunt buffalo on the eastern plains, both for food and hides; they could ride much farther afield to collect game and native plants and to trade with other tribes; and much to the chagrin of the settled Spanish colonists and Pueblo tribes, they could more effectively raid their stores of food and wares.

Before the advent of horses, Ute families lived in two kinds of seasonal shelter. In winter they occupied domed willow shelters covered with juniper bark and grass. During the summer hunting and gathering season they took shelter in wickiups, conical shelters made with brush that were supported by a framework of inner poles. Once they acquired horses and were able to procure buffalo and elk hides, they used tepees whose poles and hides could be transported from camp to camp on their mounts.

The hunting-gathering way of life continued until the Ute were forced onto reservations. With the signing of each new treaty during the late 1800s, their landholdings were diminished.

In the 1830s trapper Warren Ferris recorded in his diaries how "Women and children are employed in gathering grasshoppers, crickets, ants, and various other insects for food, together with roots and grass seed. From the mountains, they bring the nuts which are found in the cones of the pine, acorns from dwarf oaks, different kinds of berries, and the inner bark of the pine, which has a sweet and acid taste, not unlike lemon syrup. In the meantime the men are actively employed in hunting small mammals" (Pettit 1990).

Much of the Ute's medicine was derived from concoctions of wild plants. Women collected and administered herbs and other plants for healing or curing. As many as three hundred different plants have a therapeutic connection among Ute Mountain Ute.

Fibers from several plant parts, including big sagebrush bark, juniper bark, and yucca leaves, were twisted to manufacture rope and other cordage. In northern areas where the shrub was prevalent, sagebrush bark had additional applications:

BIG SAGEBRUSH
pg. 191

twined bark was used for leggings, for women's skirts, and for a poncholike shirt.

THREELEAF SUMAC
pg. 171

Willow and threeleaf sumac traditionally were woven into coiled baskets. Willow branches were cut and stored for making coarser baskets, but when the objective was to design an especially fine-quality basket, straight, pliable threeleaf sumac limbs were selected. Threeleaf sumac is often called squawbush because women were the basketmakers among the Ute, as they are among most other Indians who occupied the West.

Cactus leaves and cactus juice were employed to temper coiled clay pottery, while vegetable dyes were used to decorate animal-skin clothing. Body pigments were concocted from earth rather than from vegetable dyes. After being tanned, leather often was smoked with specific plants to impart specific colors: greasewood for a yellow hue, willow for brown, and pine for light yellow.

GREASEWOOD
pg. 149

Hunting bows, typically bent into a double-curve shape, were crafted from mountain-mahogany or juniper; less stout willow branches often were used to make single-curved training bows for young boys. Straight-grained green wood from Utah serviceberry, wild rose, or threeleaf sumac was preferred for fashioning arrows, and occasionally composite arrows were made with reed mainshafts and hardwood foreshafts.

MOUNTAIN-
MAHOGANY
pg. 165

UTAH
SERVICEBERRY
pg. 159

In contrast to the Ancestral Puebloans and contemporary Puebloans, and even the Navajo, the Ute Mountain Ute have never taken up farming as a principal way of life. Although a few families were raising garden plots planted with corn just before the reservation period, the Ute maintained a primarily hunting-gathering economy much longer into modern times than any of the other tribes living in the Four Corners region and indeed longer than most other tribes throughout the United States. Despite repeated urging by the U.S. Bureau of Indian Affairs in the 1930s and earlier, Ute were reluctant to develop farming, preferring to raise sheep or cattle. While the tribe today is experimenting with farming on a small scale, their traditions seem not to support wide acceptance of it.

Confining tribal land ownership to a reservation of some 500,000 acres has been devastating to the Ute Mountain Ute's

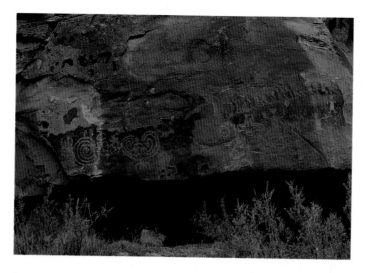

Ancestral Puebloan petroglyphs, Ute Mountain Tribal Park.

traditional way of life. Ethnographer Jan Pettit observed: "After being confined to reservations, the fearless, active men who had formerly spent their time hunting, fishing, clearing the campsite, gathering tepee poles, butchering meat, making rope, building fires, and supplying tools and other necessities for their families were obliged to become sedentary. The warrior exchanged his healthful tepee for an overheated cabin, and his diet of fresh meat, berries, and seeds, loaded with vitamins and minerals, was replaced by flour and salted meat. There were noticeable changes in the Utes' physical condition. Many Utes no longer had ambition or energy, but instead brooded on the past and became bitter" (Pettit 1990).

In recent years the tribe, now numbering nearly two thousand, has begun to develop the Ute Mountain Tribal Park, where visitors can take guided tours of some of the best-preserved Ancestral Puebloan ruins in the Southwest. More than twice as large as Mesa Verde National Park and located just south of it on the Mancos River watershed, this park also features an array of petroglyph and pictograph sites, both ancient and early historic, and generally spectacular scenery. Tourism

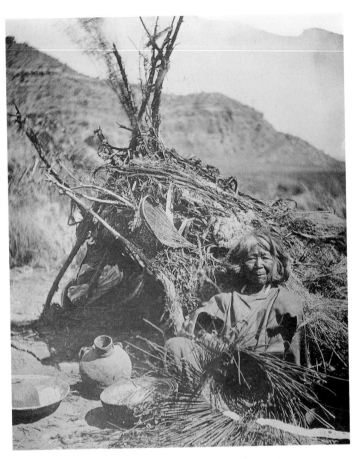

Paiute woman making basket, about 1870. Powell Expedition photograph.

(especially casino gambling) is the main source of tribal revenue today, along with gas and oil production and cattle ranching.

Two closely related Indian tribes have ties with the Four Corners region. The Southern Ute Reservation in southern Colorado adjoins and extends eastward from Ute Mountain Ute land. With about half the population of the Mountain Ute, the story of these people and their uses of wild plants closely parallels that of their neighbors.

The Southern Paiutes also have a similar background and history of wild plant use. One subgroup of these people occupied land within the Four Corners region in south-central Utah and north-central Arizona up until the nineteenth century, but this land is now incorporated within the Navajo Indian Reservation. A group known as the San Juan Southern Paiutes lives among the Navajo near Tuba City, Arizona, and continues to make and sell fine baskets, especially woven water jugs. Both Southern Ute and Southern Paiute uses of wild plants are frequently cited in chapter 11.

Suggested Reading

Callaway, Donald, Joel Janetski and Omer C. Stewart
1986   Ute. In *Handbook of North American Indians*, Vol. 11, *Great Basin*, ed. by Warren L. d'Azevedo, pp. 336–367. Smithsonian Institution, Washington, D.C.

Delaney, Robert W.
1989   *The Ute Mountain Utes.* University of New Mexico Press, Albuquerque.

Kelly, Isabel T. and Catherine S. Fowler
1986   Southern Paiute. In *Handbook of North American Indians*, Vol. 11, *Great Basin*, ed. by Warren L. d'Azevedo, pp. 368–397. Smithsonian Institution, Washington, D.C.

Pettit, Jan
1990   *Utes—The Mountain People.* Johnson Publishing Co., Boulder.

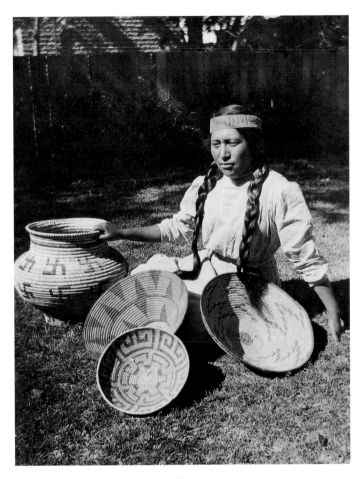

Jicarilla Apache woman with baskets, ca. 1900.

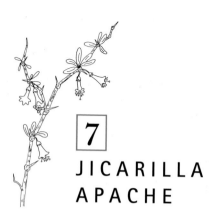

7

JICARILLA APACHE

APACHE INDIAN CULTURE and language are similar to that of the Navajo; thus, both groups are considered to have derived from the same ethnic stock. The Apache's ancestral predecessors are thought to have arrived in the New World by way of the Bering Strait land bridge, as did the Navajo's ancestors. This occurred roughly twelve to fourteen thousand years ago during the second migratory wave from Asia and before the more recent coming of the Eskimos. Anthropologists conclude that these Athapaskan-speaking Indians occupied the open plains and forests well north of the present-day United States for many millennia.

When the Apache finally moved south onto the Great Plains five hundred or more years ago, they separated into distinct groups, one of which eventually was designated Jicarilla Apache. The Spanish word may refer to a local landmark, although many believe that it translates into "little basket maker."

By this time the mammoths, the giant ground sloths, and other members of the late Pleistocene megafauna were long

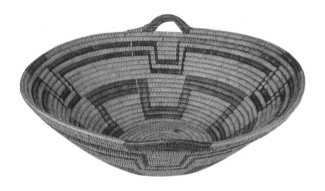

Jicarilla Apache laundry basket made from threeleaf sumac with synthetic organic dye, ca. 1920.

gone from North America, but the smaller bison we are familiar with today were abundant on the plains along with pronghorn antelope on more arid lands. The archaeological record for subsistence by prehistoric Jicarilla Apache is scanty. During the early years following their migration, though, we are sure they were hunters and gatherers of wild plants.

Among the Jicarilla, men were the hunters and raiders and women were the gatherers of wild plants for food and medicine. Piñon nuts, acorns, juniper berries, yucca fruits, grass grains, prickly pear pads, and various fruits were among the wild plant food staples still in use when Anglos entered the region in the mid-1800s. This we know from journal entries made about native peoples. Few specifics about Jicarilla herbal medicine have been recorded. We do know that several years ago young boys and girls were being taught the names of and medicinal uses for many wild plants and that both men and women practiced herbal healing. Men also used to collect in the mountains wild tobacco for ritual smoking but not for medicine.

The degree to which raiding was an ingrained practice among the Jicarilla Apache before their contact with the Spanish is not known. But if they were not already raiders, they certainly became so when tempted by Spanish and adjacent

Pueblo Indian herds of livestock. Too, the Jicarilla learned, along with the Utes and various Plains tribes, that the horse offered a means of efficient methods both for traveling and hunting bison.

Pressure from the more aggressive Comanche Indians during the 1700s had forced the Jicarilla to migrate westward off the plains into more mountainous country of the northern Rio Grande watershed. But there new Spanish land grants co-opted their settlements time and again. After their lands came under the jurisdiction of the United States in 1848, American settlers aided by the U.S. Army continued to push the Jicarilla to ever less attractive locations. A treaty designating lands that were to be the Jicarilla Apache Indian Reservation was signed in 1873. However, in the next few years shifting politics and Anglo expansion resulted in several relocations of the tribal lands. Finally in 1887 the Jicarilla were allotted their present reservation in north-central New Mexico, a place of mountains and valleys with great natural beauty.

Long before the Anglo occupation of their territory, the Jicarilla Apache were growing corn and employing agricultural practices they had adopted from the Puebloans and Spanish. Corn became important in many aspects of the Jicarilla economy and in their rituals. Corn pollen soon became a sacred substance. But when the tribe was resettled for the final time in the Four Corners region on their 870,000-acre reservation, the arable land had been largely preempted by white settlers and the people turned to raising sheep and other livestock.

While to this day the Navajo tend to avoid urban areas and instead maintain a pastoral life based around their solitary hogans, nearly one-half of the 3,200 Jicarilla choose to live in and around tribal headquarters in Dulce, New Mexico.

Once the Jicarilla people were firmly established in Dulce by the 1960s, the people turned from raising livestock to a wage economy supported by rich gas and oil deposits and a bountiful supply of commercial timber. More recently, tourism has become a major source of income generated by the sale of hunting and fishing licenses and guide services, as well as by various other tourist attractions, including a large motel and restaurant. The economically vigorous tribe also owns hotel properties and land holdings outside the reservation. The Jicarilla Art and Crafts Museum in Dulce has a basketry display and an outlet where arts and crafts are sold. These items are products encouraged by the Jicarilla Arts and Crafts Industry that was formally established in 1964.

Today, most interested outsiders associate the Jicarilla with basket weaving more than with any other craft. Traditional Jicarilla baskets are exquisite and have an inherent wild plant connection as they are always woven from threeleaf sumac or split willow twigs. More than a dozen plants provide dyes, and yucca root suds are used to clean twigs and finished baskets. Piñon gum is applied to the exterior of some baskets to make them waterproof.

On a per capita basis the Jicarilla are the most financially secure of the Indian tribes living in the Four Corners region, and nearly three-quarters of their members have at least a high school education.

Suggested Reading

Tiller, Veronica E.
1983 Jicarilla Apache. In *Handbook of North American Indians*, Vol. 10, *Southwest*, ed. by Alfonso Ortiz, pp. 440–461. Smithsonian Institution, Washington, D.C.

Worcester, Donald E.
1979 *The Apaches: Eagles of the Southwest*. University of Oklahoma Press, Norman and London.

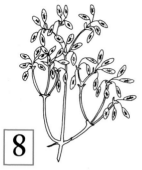

8
WEEDY GARDENS

CULTURAL REMAINS from pre-Pueblo villages of fifteen or sixteen hundred years ago present a picture of how this agrarian society developed, culminating in what we see as the Pueblo cultures of today. During the fourteenth and through the sixteenth centuries, Hopi country and the Pueblo Province comprising Zuni, Acoma, and the Rio Grande pueblos became what remain today the three major centers of Pueblo life. Indeed, most of the inhabitants of these modern villages are thought to be descendants of the Ancestral Pueblo farmers of the Four Corners.

Being the most isolated of the Puebloans, the Hopi people were least affected by Spanish and Anglo influence and imports. Perhaps it is for this reason that they appear to be the most conservative and culturally intact. Wild, semicultivated, and domesticated plants and unique, ancient gardening practices are among the many cultural artifacts they have retained. Along with their more nomadic neighbors, the Navajo, and other Puebloans to the east, the Hopi did adopt some

European fruits and vegetables from the Spanish. It has been said that they were typically eager to try new seeds and would plant anything once. The stone seed fruits such as peaches and apricots were especially prized and steadfastly cultivated in what would seem to be the most unlikely of places, the Four Corners. In this region, the Hopi are considered the model for probable prehistoric gardening techniques. This supposition is based on information provided in articles and on the fact that some Hopi still practice very old gardening techniques.

The terms agriculture, horticulture, and gardening are used here interchangeably as any method by which plants and their environment are seasonally manipulated to the benefit of a farmer and his family. Manipulation can encompass domesticated, cultivated, semicultivated, and encouraged wild plants. Agriculture, in the popular sense, assumes farming with a plow on a scale somewhat larger than gardening and includes raising of animals for food and work. Little of this applies to prehistoric farming in the Four Corners. Turkeys and dogs were the only domesticated animals known to the ancient farmers; stone hoes and fire-tempered digging sticks the only tools.

Botanical studies of contemporary Pueblo gardens demonstrate that certain wild plants are not only common on or about these gardens but that modern Indian growers deliberately introduce wild weedy annuals into their plots. As their ancestors did centuries ago, they encourage these plants by semicultivation, that is, by loosening the soil and pulling up or chopping unwanted weeds while at the same time allowing the encouraged species to share the sunlight, extra water, and nutrients in the gardens. Progeny of these wild plant species growing in old or contemporary pueblo gardens can be indicator plants of prehistoric water and soil catchments and indirectly of prehistoric gardens in the neighborhood.

Referred to as biological weeds, these plants may be introduced from thousands of miles away or be native species from the region. Whatever their origin, they are evolutionary and ecologically adapted to survive in habitats that humans have inadvertently provided for them throughout millennia of constant interaction. Because of this reciprocal plant-people

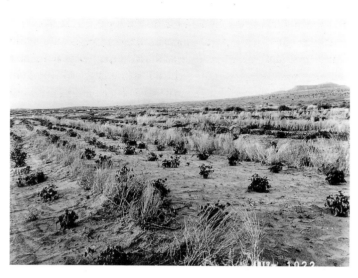

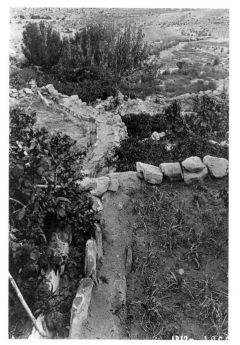

TOP
Hopi beanfield with twig rows to prevent erosion, 1935.

LEFT
Hopi terraced gardens with stone-lined irrigation channels, 1935.

relationship, these weedy species have adapted so well to the environment that they are able to remain and propagate in old fields and gardens without direct assistance from gardeners who have long since moved on.

Interestingly, quite a few of these wild, garden-indicator plants are members of the potato family (*Solanaceae*), which includes the southwestern New World wild potato (*Solanum* spp.), wolfberry (*Lycium* spp.), and groundcherry (*Physalis* spp.). Among the Old World *Solanaceae* are the contemporary garden plants, petunias, eggplant, and matrimony vine.

WOLFBERRY
pg. 180

Although geographer Carl Sauer refers to weeds among cereals crops in the following quote, his observations are equally applicable to weeds among Southwest gardens:

> The ancestors of most New World seed plants appear to have been attractive weeds. They were not tenacious intruders that the cultivator had difficulty in getting rid of, nor are they such as grow on trodden ground. They were gentle, well-behaved weeds that liked the sunshine, loose earth, and plant food of the tilled spaces, and had no great root system. Such volunteers, usable by man, were first tolerated, then protected, and finally planted (Sauer 1952).

ROCKY MOUNTAIN
BEEPLANT
pg. 222

Rocky Mountain beeplant, wild tobacco, amaranth, purslane, and others are not the stoic weeds that grow on or around prehistoric ruins but tender annuals that prefer recently disturbed or fertilized soils. In the Four Corners region, wild tobacco (*Nicotiana attenuata*) tends to germinate and grow profusely following a fire. A few years ago after wildfires at Mesa Verde, wild tobacco grew freely in the burned area and then phased out as the burn recovered and the more competitive species got a foothold. Even today, Hopi sow wild tobacco seed mixed with ash. Likewise, beeplant has appeared in abundance where none had grown for years after the flooding of old Pueblo fields on the Rio Grande. These two plants, respectively, thrived on the nutrient flush of burned vegetation ash and the dropping of silt from sluggish, muddy floodwater.

Throughout the West, wildfire is the great disrupter of vegetational stability and can result in a temporary increase of

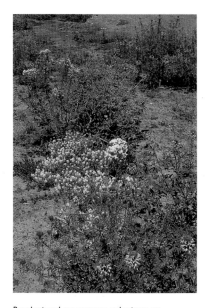

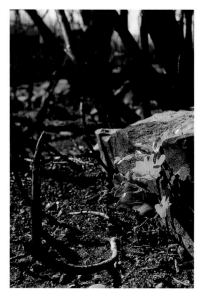

Beeplant and peppergrass, volunteers on disturbed soil.

Gambel oak sprouting shortly after the 1996 Mesa Verde fire.

local plant diversity. In August 1996, after a prolonged drought, a lightning strike started the largest forest fire in the ninety-year history of Mesa Verde National Park, virtually eliminating the piñon-juniper woodland over 4,750 acres. By late autumn, wild grasses had germinated and completely burned oak shrubs were beginning to sprout within the fire zone. We can predict that wild tobacco and several weedy plants such as peppergrass and tansy mustard will be among the first to colonize the blackened slopes.

PEPPERGRASS
pg. 219

Hereditary influence, or genetic control, is far greater for plants that have been cultivated for a long time than for species that have only recently come into cultivation. Ancient crops, cultivated and carefully selected for generations, usually produce a wealth of different varieties and forms, as with purple, white, and brown-speckled beans and red, blue, dented, flint, and sweet corn. Both corn and beans have hundreds of varieties. Wild weedy native plants that have only recently been semicultivated, such as beeplant and wild tobacco, are not highly selected or domesticated. Nevertheless, because of inherited traits, they require disturbed areas with richer soil, and are therefore more influenced by the environment than are their totally wild relatives that come up nearly anywhere.

WILD BUCKWHEAT
pg. 202

Then there are the more hardy useful native weeds such as wild buckwheat, wild potatoes, and groundcherry, all of which may still grow on old gardens or prehistoric sites where they were encouraged hundreds of years ago. Having identified these hardier garden weeds, some ethnobotanists seek to identify prehistoric fields indirectly by their plant associations. The fields themselves may have been destroyed by water erosion or wind-deposited sand dunes but they tend to be in areas that running water would have reached naturally or in the vicinity of devices to direct water or hold soil. Some weedy relics in this complex are called indicator plants and are thought, in these cases, to point to prehistoric gardens. (See *Wild Plants of the Pueblo Province* for a full discussion of indicator plants.)

Archaeologist Joseph Winter has proposed that nearly one hundred of the hardy, weedy native southwestern plants have changed in some adaptive way over thousands of years in response to constant human manipulation (Winter 1974). In our scenario, plant manipulation and management include gathering, sowing, cultivating, and sometimes burning by gardeners. The latter is a method used to encourage useful annuals, fertilize the soil, clear land, or to stimulate the pliable new growth of shrubs for basketry material. Two of these manipulated plants might be threeleaf sumac, managed by burning, and tansy mustard, managed by sowing. Some ethnobotanists have proposed that certain weedy plants were introduced in aboriginal times from Mexico along with the true domesticates—corn, beans, squash, cotton, and bottle gourd. Whether one agrees with this theory or not, it is obvious that consideration by both the gatherer and gardener has produced a unique useful weed complex that frequents middens (prehistoric dumps), village ruins, old fields, gardens, and wetlands. This brings us to the question of what constitutes a truly domesticated plant.

THREELEAF SUMAC
pg. 171

TANSY MUSTARD
pg. 216

Wild plant species grown and cared for by people do not automatically become domesticated. Wild plants remain wild even when the conditions under which they are grown greatly improve their development and yield. A genuinely domesticated plant always differs from its wild ancestor in hereditary characteristics. Gene mutations occur in all organisms, but when the resulting new characteristics are not advantageous to the plant under natural conditions, the plant does not survive. Occasionally, such traits of a plant as larger seeds or fleshier fruit are advantageous to the gatherer or farmer. By selecting those plants perceived to have favorable characteristics, growing them year after year, and saving the seed from the "best" each year, cultivated species accumulate more and more attributes favorable to the farmer but usually unfavorable for survival in the wild. The selection for larger fruit usually results in softer, juicier, thin-skinned fruit with fewer but larger seeds. Some varieties of squash are characterized by their rind: that with thin skin is harvested in summer; that with thick rind is harvested in autumn. Fruit selected for autumn harvesting, such as pumpkins, have large, protein-rich seeds as well as ample firm flesh, or marrow.

"The tendency to develop giant cells already exists among wild plants," observes one biologist. "Man has only to select the suitable forms from the wild plants accessible to him" (Schwanitz 1966). Generally, these enlarged cells are developed because of a hereditary phenomenon called gigantism. Plant gigantism is usually the result of an enlargement or multiplication of the genetic material within the cells. As a rule, this increase in the genetic material greatly increases the size of the cell. Selecting for enlarged cells holds for flowers, roots, leaves, seeds, and stems — any plant parts a gardener wishes to increase in size. While choosing varieties of plants for succulence may appease human tastes, it also makes for a plant that is more vulnerable to insects and disease. Some highly selected plants become unable to reproduce without the aid of the grower. Such is the case with the maize plant, which has all of its seeds on a cob that is tightly wrapped in a strong husk.

Prehistoric farmers of the Four Corners did not domesticate any plants from scratch except, perhaps, the dye sunflower. But they did select for different varieties of corn and beans, many of which still survive. Some special traits accumulated through thousands of years of selective breeding include the ability to flourish at this latitude, require less water, and prosper in a shorter growing season. Some beans, for instance, originated as tropical perennials. They have come a long way.

Ancestral Puebloan gardening or horticultural techniques varied depending upon where they were applied. Mesa Verdeans farmed primarily in a piñon-juniper woodland, while Chacoans did so in a desert shrubland. Canyon de Chelly provided a riparian habitat within the canyon and piñon-juniper woodland on mesa tops. These different conditions determined what gardening techniques were employed.

Core samples from old fields at Mesa Verde revealed layers of charcoal overlaid with soil containing cultigens and garden weed pollen. Some archaeologists suspect that farmers there used the swidden, or slash-and-burn, technique on their mesas to clear forests and fertilize the soil with ash. Slash-and-burn field crops flourish for only one or two years and then produce exponentially decreasing yields thereafter. The farmer must let the field rest and rejuvenate itself while he cultivates another area. Edible garden weeds such as amaranth, native wild purslane (*Portulaca retusa*), and goosefoot would have persisted for several years after the abandonment. Shrubs with edible berries, such as currants and threeleaf sumac, frequently take over a burned open-field habitat, while Gambel oak, with its nutritious acorns, colonizes a field from the edges. Therefore, even though an agricultural area may have been left fallow, it was still producing food while the farmer was slashing and burning other land in preparation for growing cultivated crops.

AMARANTH
pg. 205

PURSLANE
pg. 210

The pollen record at Mesa Verde definitely shows that as the fields advanced, the forests retreated. Recent entomological studies indicate that grasshoppers are absent from climax forests. Coprolites from Mesa Verde suggest that grasshoppers were eaten, but if the farmers themselves preferred to eat their crops, an effective way to control grasshoppers would have been with turkeys. Sure enough, archaeological remains confirm that turkeys' numbers increased over time as the clearings were enlarged on those mesas.

It is probable that such features as Mummy Lake at Mesa Verde were cisterns for holding domestic water, but also they may have held water used to irrigate mesa-top gardens, either by a ditch system or by "pot irrigation." Certainly enough pot rests have been found in ruins to suggest that some were used to steady round pots on the floor of houses and others to steady and soften the burden of ollas (water pots) on the heads of women as they carried water to the home or carried water to individual garden plants.

There is no indication that any deliberate manuring of gardens took place or that the concept of soil fertilization was even known to any of these early southwestern people. It seems doubtful, though, since so many desiccated feces have been found in the room blocks and in nearby middens.

Most of the farming at Mesa Verde was on top of the mesas, which usually received sufficient rainwater in summer and snowmelt in spring for dry farming. With the exception of cisterns, no other water source exists on mesa tops. Valleys and canyons were for the most part too narrow and dark to grow crops in, but there was some terracing on the sides of canyons with a southern or southwestern exposure.

Since Chaco Canyon receives on the average only about eight inches of precipitation a year, farming strategies had to be entirely different from those at Mesa Verde. It is unlikely that any deliberate burning was done in Chaco. Saltbush, sagebrush, and greasewood may have been burned to clear a field, but these shrubs likely were saved for cooking fires. Dry farming would succeed only during wet periods; in most years, the crops needed to be watered. Here water-saving practices and water-channeling devices were used. As far as we know, irrigation in the true sense, that of building a dam upstream of the drainage, tapping off water at this higher point, and letting it flow downstream through ditches, was probably never practiced. Instead, most agriculture took place in the broad floodplains, on mesas, and in the many sandy draws. Provision was made to capture water from cisterns on the edge of the mesas. Cisterns would fill with water, and the overflow would be channeled off the mesa into a main lateral ditch that ran parallel to the cliff. From there the water flowed into smaller lateral ditches and onto fields. Stone locks that could be moved into place in the ditches to divert water have been found, and archaeologists have discovered caches of stone hoes near ancient fields. In Chaco's broad main canyon and side canyons, rows of stones were strategically placed to slow the floodwater and catch soil and nutrient-rich plant debris. Corn, beans, and squash were probably planted in the wet, sandy soil after an early spring storm. They also could have been planted earlier with the thought that the sandy soil would contain enough moisture to stimulate the seeds to germinate and sustain the plant until summer rains fell. When the channel in Chaco Wash eroded deeply below the fields, the only way to water the crops was to hand-carry the water to the plants. Eventually the stream itself went below the surface and only emerged occasionally along the wash, and this is how it appears today.

Prehistoric garden food products from Canyon de Chelly differ somewhat from those at Chaco and Mesa Verde. Ethnobotanical remains at Antelope House indicate that beans were not a very important food item. Bean consumption was eclipsed by cottonseed, which could have provided many of the proteins and fats that beans would have supplied. The Ancestral Puebloans must have been familiar with a process that destroyed or dissipated the poisonous gossypium that cottonseeds contain. At Antelope House the main vegetable diet was not the famous triad of corn, beans, and squash but rather a combination of corn, cottonseed, cactus, beeplant, and squash.

Modern Hopi still use ancient farming methods that help us locate ancient agricultural sites and give us a sense of how their ancestors farmed. Dry farming has three critical limitations: ten inches of yearly rainfall, with four to six inches falling in summer; enough winter moisture or spring runoff to start crops; and a growing season of no fewer than one hundred and twenty days (Winter 1974). Hopi agriculture, which is marginal at best, probably yields no crops if the growing season or

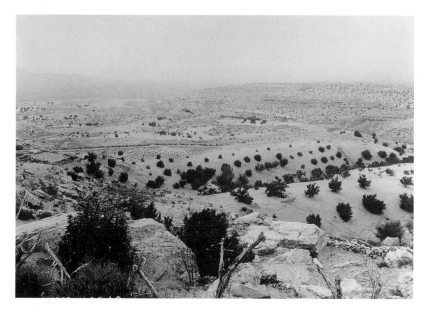

Hopi peach orchard on sand dunes, 1935.

yearly rainfall fall below these minimal conditions. Dry-farming conditions are considered good by the Hopi when all these criteria are met.

Like Ancestral Puebloans, Hopi have labored under the constant threat of food shortage. How do the Hopi, who have farmed for centuries under these minimal farming conditions, manage? Some of their responses to the specter of hunger are predictable, others ingenious.

With the exception of the slash-and-burn technique, Hopi use all of the prehistoric gardening methods previously discussed: terraces, floodwater farming, damp-soil planting, irrigation, pot irrigation, water diversion, and adding ash to sown seed. And they have added a few innovations that are probably their own. Each Hopi family tries to store one or two years' worth of food and garden seed. They plant continuously from the start of the growing season until the summer solstice to protect themselves from crop loss due to spring flooding, spring drought, or frost. Small terrace gardens tucked in and about the

Hopi mesas are hand-watered from springs at the foot of the mesas. Here, they now grow special items such as tobacco, bee-balm, onions, and melons.

The most innovative technique was developed for sand dune gardening. Sand dunes have the property of retaining moisture deep within and only giving up that moisture when it is drawn up by thirsty plant roots. So the Hopi developed a corn that is short in stature but has a root system that emerges immediately from the seed and drives downward to a depth of eight feet or more. This seed can be planted a foot or more in depth; the strength of its growing tip enables it to emerge in a day or two through sand depth impenetrable to other varieties of nonnative corn. In addition to Hopi corn, small peach and apricot trees also are grown in sand dune gardens.

SUNFLOWER
pg. 258

Sunflowers are the only wild plants that were domesticated prehistorically and are still under cultivation in the United States. The Hopi have domesticated a variety of sunflower primarily for its dye-yielding seeds, which are also edible. Although this sunflower seems to have been a historic phenomenon, its development, as well as that of the purple dye bean, reveals that little water and labor-intensive gardening have never daunted the aesthetics of Hopi gardeners.

Suggested Reading

Anderson, Edgar
1952   *Plants, Man and Life*. Little, Brown & Co., Boston.

Colton, Harold S.
1974   *Hopi Ethnobotany and Archaeological History*.
Garland Publishing, Inc. New York.

Heiser, Charles O.
1973   *Seed to Civilization*. Harvard University Press, Cambridge.

Nabhan, Gary Paul.
1989   *Enduring Seeds: Native American Agriculture and Wild Plant Conservation*. North Point Press, San Francisco.

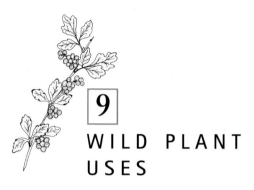

9

WILD PLANT USES

ORE THAN THREE THOUSAND species of plants are known to grow in the wild in New Mexico alone; that number climbs another thousand or so when all Four Corners states are included. Except for plants that are so tiny that they are likely to be overlooked or those that are relatively rare, a large percentage of species on these state lists are likely to have been used by people of the past, although not all uses have been documented. In this chapter we examine the principal categories of the plant uses themselves. In chapter 11, "Plants and Plantcraft," we focus on some of the most prominent species associated with native human use in the Four Corners region.

In many cases a single plant species has been used in the same manner by all or nearly all the Indian groups represented in this book. Thus, piñon pine nuts are known to have been collected for the larder during Archaic and Ancestral Puebloan times, and the nuts continue to be sought by virtually all Indian tribes living in the Southwest, as well as by many modern

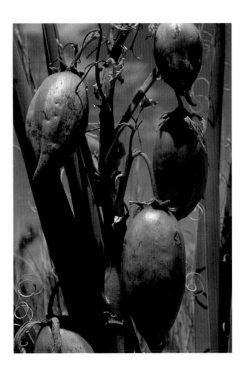

Banana yucca fruits served as food, but the roots are poisonous.

Hispanics and Anglos. The fact that at least two-thirds of the plants that have been sought by natives of the Four Corners region also have been used by Rio Grande Pueblo Indians (Dunmire and Tierney 1995) attests to the universality of plant use.

Others of these plants accrued very different uses among native peoples. For example, fourwing saltbush fruits seem to have been a food staple and the limbs an important fuelwood in prehistoric times. Later, Rio Grande Puebloans utilized the wood to make arrow points, the Navajo still use it to dye wool yellow and for medicinal applications, and the Hopi incorporate saltbush ashes as an alkali to maintain the hue from their blue cornmeal that is processed into blue piki bread. Some plants, however, were used by only a single group or clan of Indians.

Often, utility is limited to specific plant parts. Globe-mallow (*Sphaeralcea* spp.) fruit and seeds were a prehistoric food

FOURWING
SALTBUSH
pg. 152

GLOBE-MALLOW
pg. 231

item as well as used more recently by the Hopi and Southern Paiute. Its ground leaves have been used by Pueblo Indians as medicine to treat headaches and stomach problems and by the Navajo for tobacco. Globe-mallow roots have many medicinal applications, including treatment for diarrhea, colds, and sores; and powdered root skin once was associated with paint making among some native people.

In a few cases, one part of a plant may be edible and another toxic. Yucca blossoms and fruits are edible and have served as food for many in the past. This plant's root, however, with its high concentration of saponin, a toxic glucoside, is not edible. In fact, ingesting yucca root can result in a swift bout of vomiting.

YUCCA
pg. 145

Among the many categories of plant use, plants with a medicinal application are most numerous. Plants used for food rank second, while plants for concocting dye and paint rank third. In this chapter, the following categories of uses are discussed: food and beverage, medicine, construction and fuel, implements and ceremonial objects, baskets and cordage, textiles, and paints and dyes.

Food and Beverage

As discussed earlier, studies of coprolites and pollen grains at Antelope House in Canyon de Chelly have yielded a wealth of new information on Ancestral Puebloan diets. There, as at many other sites occupied during this prehistoric era, studies confirmed that corn and, secondly, squash were the dietary mainstays. The famous corn–beans–squash triad, once thought to have defined the basic diet of the time, was not supported by the evidence. Throughout most Ancestral Puebloan territory, beans apparently were never as important as corn. One of the principal researchers at Antelope House characterized the Ancestral Puebloan diet as "corn and whatever else was handy" (Morris 1986).

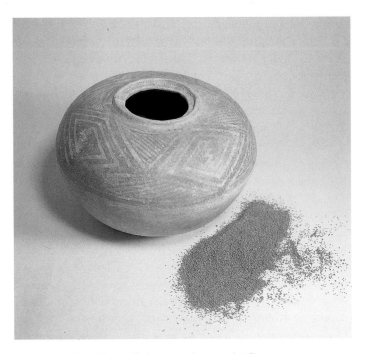

Seed pot containinig whitestem blazing star seeds recovered at Chaco.

The "handy" other food plants to which Morris referred would have varied from season to season. Cool-season grasses such as needle-and-thread grass and Indian ricegrass, along with spring-blooming perennials such as Mariposa lily and wild onion and the annual tansy mustard supplied leafy greens, starchy bulbs, and seed nourishment in the spring, a critical time of year when food stores were low and few other wild plants had yet matured. After early summer rains, edible weedy plants such as goosefoot, pigweed, and beeplant are likely to have volunteered from the wild and then became established and even encouraged either on ground that was under cultivation or on other disturbed sites around human habitations that offered a suitable niche.

A succession of other wild plants was harvested when they ripened in summer and fall. The collection of fruiting cactus and peppergrass (*Lepidium montanum*) would have been fol-

INDIAN RICEGRASS
pg. 194

MARIPOSA LILY
pg. 199

TANSY MUSTARD
pg. 216

PEPPERGRASS
pg. 219

lowed by the gathering of seeds from blazing star (*Mentzelia* spp.) and wild buckwheat (*Eriogonum* spp.) or the bulbs of wild onion or Mariposa lily. Toward summer's end, berries from shrubs and trees were at hand, among them chokecherries, wild currants, and snowberries. In good years, acorns from several species of oak and, finally, nuts from piñon cones would have been eaten or roasted and possibly stored for winter. Through much of the year, the common meal seems to have been prepared from ground ingredients that were probably mixed together and either simmered or toasted (Morris 1986).

BLAZING STAR
pg. 228

CHOKECHERRY
pg. 139

SNOWBERRY
pg. 183

PIÑON PINE
pg. 123

Corn would provide plenty of calories, but it is deficient in a number of essential nutrients, notably iron. Additionally, certain acids found in corn inhibit the absorption of this essential nutrient. Childhood illnesses and bone-growth problems have been detected from examining skeletal remains from this period, and these problems probably stem from a heavy dependence on corn (El-Najjar 1986). Iron intake from various wild plant sources such as beeplant and goosefoot would have helped counteract the iron deficiency.

ROCKY MOUNTAIN
BEEPLANT
pg. 222

GOOSEFOOT
pg. 206

Some nutrients found in wild plant foods are protein in purslane, wild buckwheat, and cactus seeds; Vitamin A in beeplant, prince's plume, purslane, and peppergrass seeds; Vitamin C in cactus stems and fruits and sagebrush leaves; potassium in peppergrass seeds and piñon nuts; and iron in most edible plant greens as well as sunflower seeds.

PRINCE'S PLUME
pg. 213

PURSLANE
pg. 210

Of course, consuming a balanced diet replete with essential nutrients was probably not a conscious endeavor among prehistoric people, but they may have recognized that those who supplemented their standard diet of corn and squash with a variety of wild plants lived longer.

The vegetarian fare was supplemented with meat from wild animals, especially rodents and rabbits as well as mule deer, pronghorn antelope, and other wild game. Although wild turkeys were domesticated early on and were raised primarily for their feathers, they were another source of meat, as were domesticated dogs. While animal meat comprised a much smaller portion of their diet than did plant foods, it certainly contributed to the essential nutrient mix.

Cows and goats were not introduced in the area until historic times, and in fact no milkable domestic animals whatsoever existed in prehistoric times here. Ancestral Puebloan people along with all other American Indians are among many ethnic groups whose bodies beyond infancy fail to produce much lactase, the enzyme needed to digest milk. Thus, even if milk had been available, the ancients probably would not have tolerated it at first. Calcium was instead provided by leafy green plants.

As noted earlier, the native peoples who make their homes in the Four Corners region today rely less and less on wild plant foods. Other than piñon nuts, still sought by everyone, it seems, wild plant gathering is more of a hobby for a few than the necessity it once was. Navajo families, many of whom still live far from urban areas, probably have maintained a greater interest in year-round plant collecting than other people of the Four Corners. However, in the cooler regions where the Ute, Paiute, and Jicarilla Apache live, picking fruits from chokecherry or other wild shrubs remains a tradition practiced by many in the fall.

Long before "regular" tea or coffee was imported into the region, people had discovered that hot beverages brewed from wild plant parts could brighten their lives, and this tradition has continued into the present. Tea brewed from the dried leaves and flowers of the Indian tea plant (*Thelesperma* ssp.) makes a vivid golden-colored, delicious hot beverage that is relished by contemporary native peoples and by many others. The aromatic leaves of the wild mint, or bee-balm (*Monarda menthaefolia*), are still sought for brewing tea, and throughout the region a cold beverage is regularly made from the berries of threeleaf sumac, otherwise called "lemonade-bush."

INDIAN TEA
pg. 256

THREELEAF SUMAC
pg. 171

Beverages concocted from juniper twigs and berries or sagebrush leaves are more likely to have been drunk for medicinal purposes than for pleasure. The same also may be true for joint-fir (*Ephedra* spp., also known as Mormon tea), and some swear by the hot beverage that can be brewed from the twigs of this plant.

JOINT–FIR
pg. 142

A notion persists that people living in prehistoric times would have discovered new edible plants by observing the

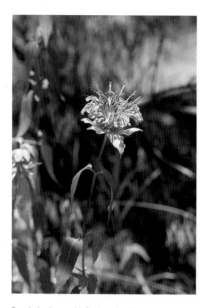

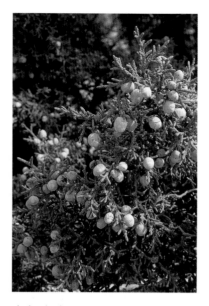

Bee–balm is sought for brewing tea.

Juniper berries were used to make a tea, probably for medicinal purposes.

habits of wild animals. This is based on the supposition that if animals eat a particular plant, it must be suitable for human consumption. While this is true for most plants, there are glaring exceptions. One of the loveliest mushrooms growing in the Great Lakes region is the colorful *Amanita muscaria*, a favorite food of red squirrels. But gatherers beware: The powerful human toxin in this mushroom could kill you.

Medicine

In sheer volume the collection of wild plants for food certainly would have exceeded that for medicinal purposes, at least in the early days. But in total number of species, many more plants growing in the Four Corners region are known for their medicinal cures. Around the world, most of the raw materials that go into the manufacture of drugs still are collected from the wild. The World Health Organization has determined that more than three-quarters of the rural populations in the world rely on an herbalist rather than on a doctor to handle their medical problems.

Most plants that eventually became useful for their medicinal properties undoubtedly were first discovered in the peoples' quest for nourishment. As we have noted, through the study of desiccated human feces, technically termed coprolites, researchers have identified with certainty many of the plants ingested by prehistoric people. This knowledge begs the question: Were the plants consumed for food or for medicinal purposes? For the answer to that question we must turn to the work of ethnobotanists who have compiled lists of hundreds of plants that have documented uses for medical treatments by various groups of Indians living in the region. When a particular species appears on several such lists (and sometimes on nearly all of them), and that plant doesn't figure strongly as a contemporary food item, it is reasonable to assume that its prehistoric use was medicinal, not culinary.

All native peoples in the Southwest have used wild plants to lessen pain, cure ailments, and improve their demeanor. Among the Ute Mountain Ute, as many as three hundred different plants were once used for their therapeutic qualities. But the Navajo seem to have made the greatest use of wild plants for medicinal purposes. Indeed, plant use is at the core of Navajo religion and central to the Navajo way of life. Among one fairly small group of Navajo, the Ramah in west-central New Mexico, an ethnobotanical study in the 1940s revealed that of the approximately four hundred wild plant species that were used by these people, more than two-thirds of them had ties to medical cures or healing ceremonial practices. For the entire Navajo Nation at least another one hundred species can be added to the medicinal plant list.

Navajo herbal medicine can be practiced in two ways. A plant or group of plants may be collected by a medicine man or woman, a clan member, or the sick person himself, although the latter practice is considered less reliable. Then an herbal tea or other concoction is made and administered to the patient along with a brief prayer. This form of treatment is usually reserved for curing more common ailments, such as colds, fevers, stomachaches, or minor injuries resulting from accidents.

For curing diseases or other major sickness or to bring about long-term good feeling or avert misfortune, herbal treatments are normally administered in a ceremony conducted by a Navajo medicine man or, less frequently, medicine woman. Medicine men and women are specialists who have undergone a long apprenticeship of training and have learned the protocols of complex ritual practices that are part of the healing ways of the Navajo people.

Harry Walters, chairperson for the Center for Diné Studies at the Navajo Community College in Tsaile, Arizona, explained to us that, in his view, sharing information about herbal medicine among the Navajo is not as restricted as it is among the Pueblo Indians, who are intent upon keeping this knowledge within their clans. In most cases, sharing such information is up to individual Navajo medicine men. Healing is their profession, and as with other doctors they are not likely to disseminate trade secrets. We have elected to steer away from discussing ceremonial or ritual uses of plants by Navajo or other native people whose traditions are discussed in this book, as it is clear that certain aspects of this kind of knowledge are sacred and not meant to be shared with outsiders.

From our own recent experience, we have noticed that some Western medical doctors occasionally are recommending the use of over-the-counter herb-based medicine, with a more than fair rate of success. This certainly is in contrast to the past when herbal medicine was an anathema to most physicians in the United States. Because we now understand the scientific basis for the success rate attributed to wild plant cures, practitioners of Western medicine are more comfortable using them.

Wild bearberry (*Arctostaphylos uva-ursi*) serves as an example. Its leaves contain arbutin, tannic and gallic acids, quercetin, and hydroquinone, all of which have antiseptic, diuretic, and

WILD BEARBERRY
pg. 177

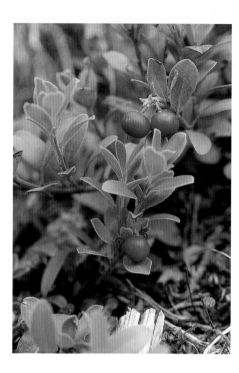

Wild bearberry has been widely used in herbal medicines.

astringent qualities. Thus, it's not surprising that bearberry is incorporated in herbal medicines to combat inflammation. Bearberry tea, available commercially, is sold throughout the world as a treatment for various bladder and kidney ailments. Interestingly, few native tribes of the Four Corners where the plant is common at higher elevations seem to have recognized it for these medicinal purposes. Across the region they did seek out this plant but rather for smoking the dried leaves as tobacco in ceremonies and for pleasure.

It has been only in the last seventy years, following the discovery of penicillin in a fungus, that pharmaceutical companies began in earnest to isolate these components. Once an effective agent from a wild plant has been chemically identified, it is usually manufactured synthetically and mass-produced with greater dosage reliability than if extracted from the plants themselves. An obvious additional benefit of synthetic manufacture is that wild plant populations are protected from over-collection.

The commercial development of modern nonprescription herbal medicines represents an alternative somewhere between medicine plant collection and use by native peoples and the costly analysis and production of drugs by the pharmaceutical corporations. These "natural" medicines have long been favored by various cultures throughout the world, especially in the Orient and Germany, to say nothing of third world countries. In the past decade the United States has experienced a ground swell of interest in these alternative medicines. Today more than one thousand homeopathic preparations are sold over the counter along with a sometimes bewildering variety of vitamins, minerals, and herbal remedies.

These products rarely have been professionally analyzed for their chemical properties. A typical label on a well-known brand bottle of health-aid tablets reads, "The extract of this product has been scientifically calibrated to ensure guaranteed levels of naturally occurring fatty acids and sterols." Yet for various ordinary ailments, these products often seem to work!

Construction and Fuel

As discussed in chapter 3, the Ancestral Puebloans who occupied Chaco Wash and surrounding locations a thousand years ago were master builders. The story of how the people cut, transported, and used large timbers at Chaco is especially fascinating because, except for cottonwoods and willows growing along the main wash, the canyon bottom is practically devoid of trees today, and the Chaco environment hasn't been truly forested for many thousands of years.

Vast quantities of wooden beams and other construction elements were used to construct hundreds of pueblos and smaller residences. For the ten largest complexes alone, this operation required the cutting with stone axes of two hundred

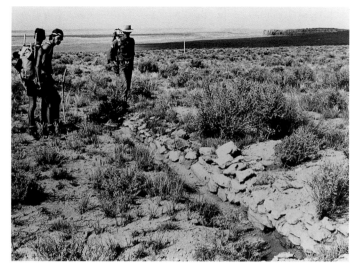

Ancient log-hauling road from Chuska Mountains to Chaco.

thousand or more trees, most of which had to be hauled in from long distances. Long-distance hauling was particularly the case for the approximately forty-five thousand spruce and fir trees used in the largest pueblos at Chaco, since spruce and fir logs could only have come from mountain ranges no closer than fifty miles from the construction sites (Betancourt et al. 1986). Straight logs of ponderosa pine were the most common wood for cutting beams here. Douglas-fir, cottonwood, and, to a lesser extent, piñon pine and juniper made up the other principal woods that were harvested for manufacturing beams.

While the people of Chaco had to travel long distances to obtain wood for house construction, especially during Chaco's later years, the people at other Ancestral Puebloan centers relied on whatever wood was available from much closer sources. For example, at Aztec and Mesa Verde there was greater use of aspen, Douglas-fir, and juniper; however, piñon pine was not employed in construction projects at Aztec (Thomas Windes, personal communication, 1996).

Karen Adams applied her considerable ethnobotanical expertise to the study of roof construction at Salmon Ruin, an outlying Chacoan great house located fifty miles to the north, and she described to us the construction sequence: "In one room at least five wooden timbers, or *vigas*, were placed across the north-south axis of the room and secured into wall sockets to form the main roof supports. Directly above, two- to three-inch tree limbs, or *latillas*, were laid across the vigas. On top of all this was a continuous layer of closely spaced willow twigs arranged cross-wise to the main series of latillas. A thick layer of adobe was packed over the branches, and this was topped by juniper bark and another layer of adobe, in turn forming the floor surface upon which a second story could be built." The fact that Chaco and Salmon Ruin are located in such dry climate zones has allowed this sequence to be preserved nearly intact for centuries.

Pueblo construction at Chaco seems to have coincided with cycles of wetter-than-average weather, suggesting that extra manpower was freed up for house building during times of food surplus. National Park Service archaeologists Tom Windes and Dabney Ford in 1985 began tracking these events at prehistoric Chaco, and their findings reveal a fascinating history in the procurement, use, and reuse of wood (Windes and Ford 1996).

The Ancestral Puebloans at Chaco satisfied most of their cooking and warming fuel needs with shrubby, nonconiferous plants, such as greasewood, fourwing saltbush, sagebrush, and rabbitbrush. This may be because piñon and juniper, the preferred fuelwoods of Four Corners natives, were not growing that extensively here, and juniper wood, especially, had much more important applications. Toward the end of the era of human habitation at Chaco, there is compelling evidence that fuelwood, as well as that for construction, was being imported from a distance. The eventual depletion of fuelwood is one of several possible reasons for the eventual abandonment of the Chaco complex.

Implements and Ceremonial Objects

The excavation of Antelope House in Canyon de Chelly in the late 1970s yielded a vast amount of information about how Ancestral Puebloans used wood to craft a variety of tools and other implements (Magers 1986b). From Pamela Magers's studies we learn that the woods from various native trees and shrubs tended to be used in specific ways, depending upon the physical characteristics of the wood.

At Antelope House and other sites of this era, threeleaf sumac and willow branches often were selected when a flexible material was needed. Willow-sumac products included snow-shoe frames, cradleboard hoops, and pot rest coils. Willow and sumac also were used as the foundation for most basketry.

WILLOW
pg. 130

When stouter wood was needed, Gambel oak or moun-tain-mahogany were obvious choices. At Antelope House, implements made from these woods included digging sticks, hoes (similar to digging sticks but with the use end flared into a blade), throwing sticks, tool handles, and various rods. Other tough, fairly straight-grained woods used for the manufacture of such items were greasewood (*Sarcobatus vermiculatus*), Utah serviceberry (*Amelanchier utahensis*), cliff fendlerbush (*Fendlera rupicola*), box-elder (*Acer negundo*), and Douglas-fir (*Pseudotsuga menziesii*). When any of the above implements required ties, the cordage invariably was made from yucca fiber, which also supplied the raw material for netting, secured with square or overhand knots, used for hoops in the hoop-and-dart game.

GAMBEL OAK
pg. 136

MOUNTAIN-
MAHOGANY
pg. 165

GREASEWOOD
pg. 149

UTAH
SERVICEBERRY
pg. 159

CLIFF
FENDLERBUSH
pg. 157

Cottonwood provided one of the softest, most easily carved materials, and it often was used for discs, stirring paddles, scoops, and fire-making equipment. A typical fire tool kit was comprised of a softwood hearth, or tablet, and a shaft. The shaft's fire-blackened and use-polished tip fit into the drilled holes of the hearth and was twirled, producing sufficient heat to ignite shred-ded juniper bark or other easily torched materials.

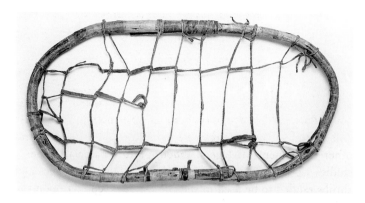

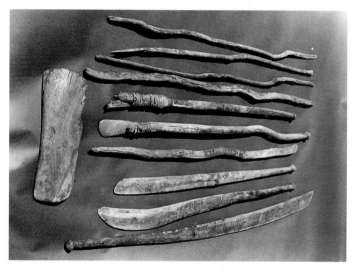

TOP
Gambel oak swinging cradle or snowshoe frame, probably Puebloan.

BOTTOM
One-thousand-year-old digging sticks and gardening tools from Chaco, made from Gambel oak, cottonwood, and willow; stone tips fastened with yucca cordage.

A variety of woods, including oak, willow, Douglas-fir, and cottonwood, were used to make bows. At Antelope House, 232 arrows and arrow fragments were recovered. The mainshafts were all crafted from common reed (*Phragmites communis*) that

COMMON REED
pg. 197

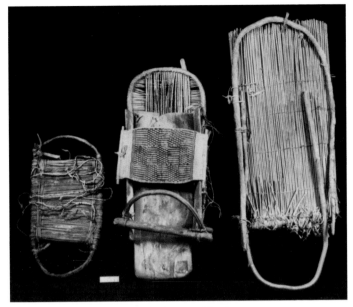

Cradles from Antelope House with oak and coyote willow frames, common reed backing, and tied with banana yucca cordage.

grew plentifully along the main wash. Eleven different woods were used to tip the arrows. Greasewood, mountain-mahogany, cliff fendlerbush, and willow were the most common materials for arrow points that were inserted into the reed stems.

Threeleaf sumac (*Rhus trilobata*) was most frequently used for prayer sticks, split dice, fetishes, objects resembling "god's eyes," and other ceremonial objects recovered here. It is clear that this plant, so useful as a source of food and for making baskets, dye coloring, and various implements, had important ceremonial connotations as well.

THREELEAF SUMAC
pg. 171

Many of these wood uses were continued by the descendants of those who occupied Antelope House and other Ancestral Puebloan sites. Modern Hopi use cottonwood drills and hearths to produce ceremonial fires. Cottonwood also is the favored raw material for making drums and for carving a host of domestic and ceremonial articles, including kachina dolls.

COTTONWOOD
pg. 133

Until the mid-1800s, Ute Indians and certainly others living in the Four Corners region were using native woods for a variety of implements: serviceberry or threeleaf sumac for snowshoe frames, and wild rose, serviceberry, or other berry woods for arrows. Ethnographer Anne Smith has described the Ute process for making bows: "The wood bow was made of cedar (juniper), chokecherry, or service berry. A suitable piece of green wood, about four feet long, was obtained and put to dry. Then the bark was scraped off with a stone and the bow was whittled. It was flat on one side, gently rounded on the other, and tapered toward either end. It was rubbed smooth with a stone. Then the wood was warmed over the fire, grease (preferably mountain sheep or deer fat) was rubbed in well, and the wood was bent and shaped over their knee.... The method of manufacture was the same for the single-curved as for the double-curved bow" (Smith 1974).

WILD ROSE
pg. 162

CHOKECHERRY
pg. 139

Baskets and Cordage

When the mammoths and other giant creatures that stalked the plains during the wane of the last glacial period died out or migrated eastward, Paleo-Indian people shifted to gathering wild plants and hunting small animals. Consequently, their basic tool kit changed as well; spears, atlatls, and stone implements used for processing large game were replaced by milling stones and basins for grinding wild seeds and by woven trays and baskets for carrying and cooking plant products.

By the time people had settled in villages and were raising domesticated corn, squash, and beans in the Four Corners region, it was the era of the Ancestral Puebloans, and basket making was a major pursuit. Indeed, the Basketmaker period, so-named by Richard Wetherill, lasted from roughly 100 B.C. through A.D. 600.

Baskets of this period are often intricately crafted and handsomely decorated. They came in many sizes and shapes,

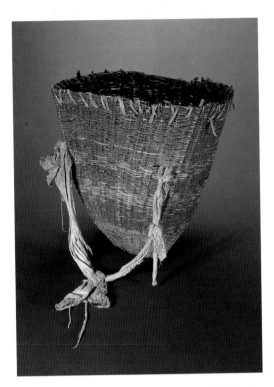

Hopi burden basket plaited with threeleaf sumac and reinforced
with Utah juniper rods, ca. 1880–1910.

RABBITBRUSH
pg. 188

PIÑON PINE
pg. 123

and most were woven from willow, threeleaf sumac, yucca, rabbitbrush, reed, or cattails. Woven baskets were waterproofed by
lining them inside and out with piñon pine pitch. Such baskets
could be used as cooking vessels by dropping hot stones into
the water they contained. Still, when pottery making was introduced from the south before the time of Christ, fewer basket
were needed.

Basket making thus declined for a time, but it was never
forgotten. Although those who moved from the Four Corners
south into the Rio Grande corridor continued to weave baskets
made from wild plant material, basket making is no longer
widely practiced among people living at the various pueblos in
New Mexico. Such is not the case for the Hopi, whose basketry

as well as pottery flourishes today. The earliest Hopi baskets that have been preserved are similar to Ancestral Puebloan–era types and typically are made from plaited yucca leaves, sometimes turned over a sumac frame at the rim. Hopi coiled baskets that are of precontact vintage tend to be in the form of trays.

Over time, clans from each of the Hopi mesas developed distinctive styles. On Third Mesa today wicker baskets are woven from yucca, sumac, or rabbitbrush; on occasion willow or wild currant is used in lieu of sumac for the foundation. Inhabitants of Second Mesa produce a coiled ware made from a core of galleta grass (*Hilaria jamesii*) stems or yucca leaves wrapped and sewn together with strips of split narrowleaf yucca leaves. Watertight coiled jars are crafted from willow splints. Traditional baskets are often decorated with yucca strips that have been colored with native plant dyes. On First Mesa the craftspeople tend to be potters rather than basketmakers. Among the Hopi, basket making is done by women, pottery making by men.

NARROWLEAF YUCCA
pg. 145

Ute Indians also are famous for their basketry. Threeleaf sumac, gathered in the spring when it is soft and supple, is preferred for the finest quality coiled baskets, while thin wands of willow might be used for coarser ware. Anne Smith describes how the Ute waterproofed a jug basket: "Pine gum was collected, melted in a kettle until it was soft, then poured into the basket, and the basket was turned around and around, so the pitch would fill up all the interstices. Small hot pebbles were put in with the pitch, and helped give a solid coating to the inside, as they were shaken around with the hot pitch....The stopper was usually a plug of sagebrush bark, sometimes attached to the neck of the bottle by a buckskin string" (Smith 1974). The art of making traditional baskets is being carried on by a few. Neomi Red, who is a Ute Mountain Ute married to a Southern Ute and who lives on the reservation at Ignacio, Colorado, told us that she is teaching her five daughters to make pitch-covered water jugs from willows growing in the wild.

THREELEAF SUMAC
pg. 171

WILLOW
pg. 130

SAGEBRUSH
pg. 191

Basket weaving is still a fine art practiced among Jicarilla Apache women, although today many of the basketmakers use

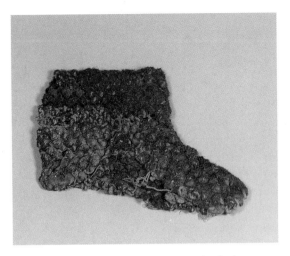

Ancestral Puebloan bootie made with yucca and turkey feathers from cave south of Blanding, Utah.

commercial dyes for coloring the split twigs. Lydia Pesata, a noted Jicarilla basketmaker who learned how to weave baskets from her husband's grandmother, has been weaving for more than thirty years, and she is one of the few who use strictly wild plant sources. Lydia explained that she prefers threeleaf sumac over willow for the base material, and said she collects wild plants year-round for dyeing the splints. She also told us that she uses suds produced by pulverized yucca roots to clean her baskets.

One of the great leaps forward for an advancing culture in pre-Ancestral Puebloan times would have been the discovery of how to make cordage from wild plant material. Long before cotton made its way north from where it was originally culti-vated in Mexico, wild plant fibers were being processed into twine. Woody fibers, called bast, from juniper and cliffrose (*Cowania stansburiana*), fibers from milkweed (*Asclepias* spp.) and dogbane (*Apocynum* spp.), as well as human and animal hair were employed in the manufacture of prehistoric textiles and twine. But fibers from banana yucca (*Yucca baccata*) and nar-rowleaf yucca (*Y. angustissima* and *Y. glauca*) leaves played the most important role in the lives of the early people. Bundles of

CLIFFROSE
pg. 168

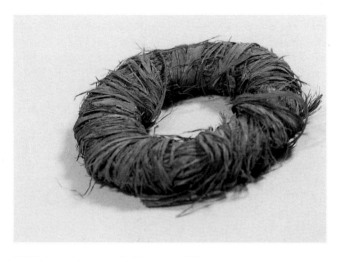

Utah juniper pot rest wrapped with yucca cord, from Mesa Verde.

split yucca leaves tied with yucca cord have regularly turned up at Archaic period cave sites and in Ancestral Puebloan ruins.

Another wild plant and prehistoric pottery connection comes from Canyon de Chelly's Antelope House. To extend the life of a damaged vessel, "the most common practice is the drilling of repair holes from the exterior of the vessel on either side of the crack or break.... Vegetal material then was wound through the holes to bind the break. Strips of *Rhus trilobata* [threeleaf sumac] were used in nine of the twelve repaired specimens with vegetal material preserved. Exploiting the good qualities of *Rhus* for a strong and tight repair probably is an extension of its use in basket making" (Schaefer 1986).

Historic accounts given by descendants who are members of the twenty southwestern Pueblo nations indicate that yucca fiber was prepared by first crushing the leaves and then separating and cleaning the fibers with a scraper. Roasting or boiling the leaves, followed by chewing them, was another method thought to have been used by Puebloans. However, a few years ago Carolyn Osborne, a researcher at Mesa Verde National Park, experimented with yucca fiber preparation and found that

YUCCA
pg. 145

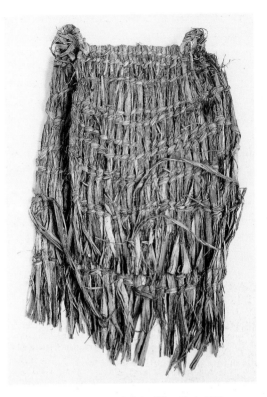

Southern Paiute girl's skirt made from cliffrose bark, 1932.

roasted yucca leaves were difficult, if not impossible, to process. She also doubts that chewing was a principal method in making the yards and yards of yucca fiber that must have been produced to meet even a single prehistoric family's needs. The method she found to be most effective for separating fiber from leaf tissue involved soaking pounded or boiled leaves in water for about a week, then using a scrapper made from bone or a flake of stone to separate the fiber from the leaf tissue. The saponin in yucca leaves makes twisting or spinning the fibers into yarn easier (Osborne 1965).

Textiles

Textiles differ from basketry in that they are made with fine, flexible materials on a loom or other device that holds the filaments in place during the weaving process. Before the introduction and cultivation of domestic cotton, the earliest prehistoric weavers of textiles had to use hair from humans, domesticated dogs, and wild animals; bird skins or feathers; or leaf and stem fibers from wild plants.

By the time that the Chacoan culture was flourishing late in the first millennium A.D., domesticated cotton plants had been imported from Mexico. At first, cotton appears to have

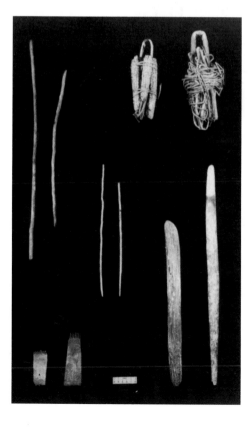

Weaving tools from Antelope House: willow and corn-cob loom anchors; cottonwood and juniper battens; greasewood and mock-orange finishing needles; cottonwood weaving combs.

been scarce in our region, and it was used sparingly. By the 1200s, soft threads from cotton bolls were the principal fibers the Ancestral Puebloans used to weave textiles. The earliest looms seem to have been a backstrap type with one end rod connected to the weaver's waist and the other to a tree or house wall. Only narrow cloths could be woven on this type of loom. The importation of cotton and the invention of a larger, upright loom meant that wider, lightweight material could now be manufactured for clothing, blankets, and other items.

Cotton growing and textile manufacturing were major occupations at Canyon de Chelly. From the excavations of Antelope House, where 95 percent of all recovered woven material was made from cotton, we also learn how wild plants were employed in spinning, weaving, and sewing (Magers 1986a).

THREELEAF SUMAC
pg. 171

CLIFF
FENDLERBUSH
pg. 157

MOUNTAIN-
MAHOGANY
pg. 165

GAMBEL OAK
pg. 136

Flexible threeleaf sumac twigs were used to make beaters for removing cotton seeds from the fluff and for loom rods. Willow, cliff fendlerbush, and a half-dozen other wild plants also went into the making of these rods used to control weaving rhythm. Battens for tightening the weave were made of mountain-mahogany, juniper, and box-elder, among other species. Buried anchors that stabilized the looms employed loops of Gambel oak, willow, or threeleaf sumac that were tied together with yucca fiber cords to form an eye hook. Yucca cord also was used for ties on looms, and sewing needles were made from the sharp-tip end of narrowleaf yucca leaves. The discovery of loom anchors and loom holes in four different Antelope House kivas supports the theory that weaving, almost surely done by men, was linked with the kivas.

When the Spanish first entered the Rio Grande Valley from Mexico in 1540, they encountered Pueblo Indians dressed in embroidered cotton garments decorated with figures in many colors. The tradition of weaving cotton into blankets and garments also was carried on by Hopi Pueblo men well into this century. Today, however, very few weavers practice their craft on the Hopi mesas.

By the time the Spanish were entrenched in the Southwest in the 1700s, the Navajo had learned all about weaving from

Puebloans (or from Spider Woman, according to their own revered stories). From then on they advanced it from a functional craft to a highly developed art form. From the start the Navajo wove not with cotton but with wool from the sheep that had been introduced a century earlier. In contrast to the Puebloans, it was the women who took up weaving. As the bearers of children, Navajo weavers often say, "the rugs are like our children." Traditional Navajo look at their weaving as an expression of the essence of being Navajo, almost comparable to a permanent written record (Paul Zolbrod, personal communication, 1996).

Before the mid-1800s, the Navajo made clothing and blankets for their own use. Although textiles were made for ceremonial purposes, after the American invasion of 1846 the weavers began to produce colorful rugs for an off-reservation market. It was not long before trading posts featuring ever-more intricately colored and finely woven rugs sprang up across the reservation. By 1889, nineteen of these posts, all licensed by the Bureau of Indian Affairs, were in operation. The interest in Navajo rugs was blooming, and it has not abated since.

Both Hopi and Navajo traditionally wash their rug wool with frothy suds whipped up from crushed yucca plant roots:

YUCCA
pg. 145

> The root of the yucca, which is about 18 inches long, is dug from the ground. It is a fibrous, tough, yellow substance, full of a rather glutinous sap. These roots are pounded with a rock until the fibers are separated and torn apart.
>
> A bowl of water is then warmed over the fire (or cold water is used) and the fibrous, pounded yucca root is placed in it and worked with the hands until a fine white suds is obtained. The yucca is then squeezed out and put away for future use. It may be used several times, after re-pounding, although the root is much more effective when fresh (Colton 1965).

Paints and Dyes

The number of different wild plant species that have been associated with creating decorative coloring for pots, textiles, and
other objects is exceeded only by those used for food and medicine.

ROCKY MOUNTAIN
BEEPLANT
pg. 222

TANSY MUSTARD
pg. 216

Ancestral Puebloan potters in the Four Corners region first
began to paint their ware around A.D. 600. A temporary rich
black was produced from a concentrate prepared by boiling the
leafy stems of Rocky Mountain beeplant (*Cleome serrulata*) or,
perhaps, yellow beeplant (*C. lutea*) that were gathered early in
summer when the plants contain high amounts of iron. Painted
designs were applied after the pot was slipped, and upon firing,
the color softened to a dark gray. Tansy mustard (*Descurainia
pinnata*) was another plant prepared in much the same way to
make black pottery paint. Both these vegetal paints have a tendency to produce slightly blurred edges on the designs, and this
blurring is diagnostic of vegetal paints.

Later in the people-pottery sequence, iron oxide pigments
from the earth, sometimes mixed with vegetal pigments, were
probably used. Other wild plants associated with ancient pottery painting include wild dock and piñon pine. It is likely no
coincidence that all these plants known to produce ceramic
pigments also happen to have edible parts. Hopi and other
contemporary Pueblo potters who have chosen to follow
traditional methods continue to use both mineral and wild
plant–based paints.

During Ancestral Puebloan times, paint was used to make
pictographs and murals and to color various wooden objects.
Images that were painted on rocks are called pictographs (as
opposed to petroglyphs, which are pecked, incised, or scratched
on rock surfaces). Although less common than petroglyphs,
pictographs still are plentiful in the Four Corners region. They
are typically applied in various shades of red or brown, less
often black, and a few are polychromatic, incorporating blue,
green, or yellow. Nearly all employ inorganic pigments proba-

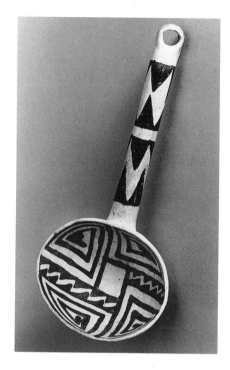

Ancestral Puebloan dipper from southern San Juan Basin, with black paint prepared from beeplant or tansy mustard, A.D. 1100–1200.

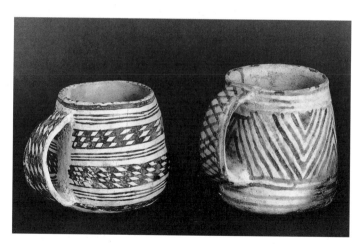

Mesa Verde mugs painted with beeplant or tansy mustard guaco, A.D. 1200–1300.

bly made from locally available minerals. These paints are relatively insoluble in water, and they have endured on the rocks for centuries. Vegetable pigments also were likely to have been used, but these tend to be water soluble and not long lasting.

Mineral-based paints also were preferred for rendering the beautiful murals that decorated the inside walls of many kivas from this era. However, at least one set of murals from a prehistoric Hopi kiva on Antelope Mesa employed vegetal paint. The black color that was used throughout these murals was often a pigment derived from wood charcoal, beeplant guaco, or, perhaps, tansy mustard (Smith 1952).

A number of wooden objects with brightly painted or stained surfaces have been recovered from Ancestral Puebloan sites such as the eleventh-century Chetro Ketl ruin at Chaco (Dodgen 1978). Most of the pigments analyzed from the Chetro Ketl collection appear to have come from various mineral sources; wild plants, though, seem to have contributed to the coloration of some paints: crushed wood charcoal for black, piñon or other conifer resin for a lustrous brown, and possibly rabbitbrush blossoms for yellow. Indian paintbrush (*Castilleja linearifolia*) roots mixed with juniper bark and white clay may have been the source for a reddish-orange organic paint that was applied to some objects made from gourds. At least that has been a practice among Hopi in more recent times (Whiting 1939).

PIÑON PINE
pg. 123

RABBITBRUSH
pg. 188

JUNIPER
pg. 126

Basket making, which preceded Ancestral Puebloan pottery making by several hundred years, eventually incorporated colored splints, usually black, brown, or red, combined with the natural color of the basic material. The specific plants used to concoct a dye for the splints is unknown, as is the source for the earliest dyes applied to material woven from cotton.

Our best information on dye plants from the Four Corners region comes from the Hopi and Navajo. More than fifty species of wild plants have been associated with wool and cotton textile dyes. Among the dye plant parts most frequently sought by the Hopi are Indian tea (*Thelesperma megapotamicum*) flowers, which produce the richest and most permanent reddish-gold hues. Cliffrose twigs and leaves are employed for

INDIAN TEA
pg. 256

CLIFFROSE
pg. 168

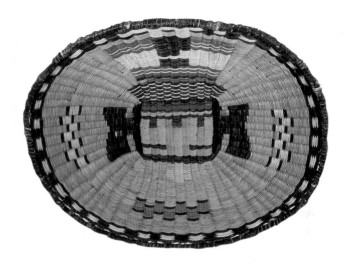

Hopi Third Mesa basket made from rabbitbrush and yucca, 1920. Black dye is from boiled sunflower seeds; light is sunbleached yucca; red is synthetic organic dye.

gold, rabbitbrush and goldenrod flowers for yellow, and steamed sunflower seeds for maroon. When sunflower seeds are mixed with yellow ocher, the dye yielded is black. The ashes from burned fourwing saltbush branches are used by Hopi to maintain the blue color present in blue cornmeal that is used to make their famous piki wafer bread.

    Navajo women collect and grind red prickly pear fruits to give white wool a rose or pink shade or mix it with a liquid from the root bark of mountain-mahogany to obtain a soft reddish tan. Ground lichens produce various colors, but, of course, many traditional Navajo rugs are undyed, the black, gray, brown, or tan colors coming directly from the sheep. The same plant species collected in different parts of the region may yield varying shades of color. Interestingly, there is not a great deal of overlap between Hopi and Navajo dye plants even though both peoples live in similar environments with nearly identical wild plant resources.

GOLDENROD
pg. 250

SUNFLOWER
pg. 258

FOURWING
SALTBUSH
pg. 152

PRICKLY PEAR
pg. 234

MOUNTAIN-
MAHOGANY
pg. 165

It is the roots of many plants that yield dye. When we met with Lydia Pesata, an expert Jicarilla Apache traditional basketmaker, she told us she likes to look for dye plants in disturbed areas. That's because roots may be close to the surface or actually exposed, staining the soil if the root has dye qualities. "That is how you discover dye plants" she said. Sure enough, during a field trip with her in the spring of 1996, we spotted two soil stains in a recent road-cut. The reddish-brown coloration was caused by the exposed roots from a nearby Gambel oak, and a yellow stain was caused by the damaged root of barberry (*Berberis fendleri*). Lydia was delighted with the find, since she isn't able to obtain much of either dye source for her baskets these days, as the roots are so difficult to dig up. Her husband carries a shovel in his pickup for just such occasions.

GAMBEL OAK
pg. 136

BARBERRY
pg. 156

By far the handiest reference for dye plant recipes attributed to craftspeople living in the Four Corners region comes to us from a neat little book, *Navajo and Hopi Dyes*. Recently published (but undated) by Bill Rieske, it is a combined reprinting of two long out-of-print publications, *Navajo Native Dyes* (Bryan and Young 1940) and *Hopi Dyes* (Colton 1965).

Suggested Reading

Ayensu, Edward S.
1981   A Worldwide Role for the Healing Powers of Plants. *Smithsonian* 12(8):87–97.

Kent, Kate Peck
1983   *Prehistoric Textiles of the Southwest*. School of American Research Press and University of New Mexico Press, Albuquerque.

1985   *Navajo Weaving: Three Centuries of Change*. School of American Research Press, Santa Fe.

Mayes, Vernon O. and Barbara Bayless Lacy
1989   *Nanisé : A Navajo Herbal*. Navajo Community College Press, Tsaile, AZ.

Moore, Michael
1989   *Medicinal Plants of the Desert and Canyon West.*
Museum of New Mexico Press, Santa Fe.

Sauer, Carl O.
1952   *Agricultural Origins and Dispersals.* Bowman Memorial
Lectures, Series 2. The American Geographical Society, New
York.

Tierney, Gail D.
1977   Plants for the Dyepot. *El Palacio* 83(3):28–35.

Whiteford, Andrew Hunter, Stewart Peckham, Rick
Dillingham, Nancy Fox and Kate Peck Kent
1989   *I Am Here: Two Thousand Years of Southwest Indian Arts
and Culture.* Museum of New Mexico Press, Santa Fe.

Willink, Roseann S. and Paul G. Zolbrod
1996   *Weaving a World: Textiles and the Navajo Way of Seeing.*
Museum of New Mexico Press, Santa Fe.

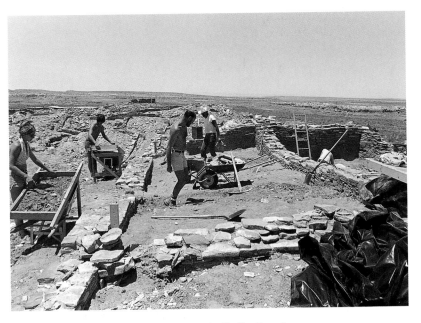
Modern archaeologists excavating at Pueblo Alto, Chaco Canyon.

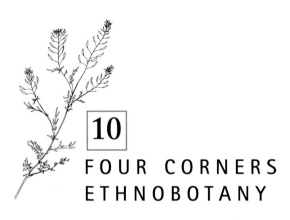

10

FOUR CORNERS ETHNOBOTANY

ETHNOBOTANY IS THE STUDY of how people use native plants. It is a dual science concerned with plants and the wisdom of people who use them. Without realizing it, people all over the world have been practicing ethnobotany ever since the first human beings communicated information about plants to one another. They told each other what plants were poisonous, sweet, or medicinal and which could be used as food or was worth the energy to obtain and process it. Plants contribute much to the very essence of humanity, our culture. Indirectly, by investigating the botanicals people use we learn something about how they interacted with nearly all other aspects of their natural environment, including the fauna, landforms, soil, climate, seasons, and even the sky.

In the Four Corners, Indian peoples and plants have had a long and reverential relationship. The Hopi and their immediate ancestors have planted, gathered, and utilized plants for at least a thousand years, while the "newcomers," the Ute, Apache, and Navajo, have amassed some six hundred years of botanical experience in this region. The antiquity of human plant use is suggested by the tiny pieces of botanicals, as well as by ancient tools and household items, which were made of plant material, found today in ruins and rock shelters and even scattered within vegetation growing upon ruins or in old fields. Kiva murals, pottery forms, baskets, stories, and structures, as well as the contemporary use of objects that are similar to ancient artifacts and the use of plants by local folks, provide clues for interpreting prehistoric materials. Increasingly, ethnobotanists seek information from their colleagues in other sciences, as well as from people of the very cultures they are studying. It has been said that "the past is the key to the future"; in ethnobotany, the present is the key to interpreting the past.

Since these interpretive approaches are directly or indirectly related to plants, a few of them are mentioned here. One of our favorites is the application of ethnoastronomy, seemingly a universe away from green plants, but its connection with ethnobotany lies in the art of divining, from celestial objects, the seasons for the proper time to plant seeds or perform the ceremonies to ensure fecundity of both plants and man. The mysterious "sun dagger" atop Fajada Butte, a singular and nearly inaccessible mesa at Chaco Canyon, was revealed, at least partially, to be the hands in the sun clock used in predicting the solstices and, indirectly, the seasons. At some pueblos certain landmarks between which the sun rises or sets determine a ritual calendar that, in turn, determines the human cycle of life: for example, when to plant, when to harvest, or when to marry.

Just as there are ceremonies for bridging the gap between the seasons, myth and lore narrow the chasm between history and prehistory. Until recently, no written language existed for any of the many southwestern Indian language groups. In the absence of written literature, the ability to pass down knowledge verbally or by example became key to cultural integrity. This oral tradition, dependent upon listening and observing, remains strong among Native American people today. Storytelling, now being transcribed into written form by Native American authors and illustrators, charms and enlightens us all. Southwest Indian tales collected years ago are not merely enjoyable, they are tradition-bearing, informative cultural artifacts. To show how this can work into modern times, we have a story to share about the solution to a problem not originally perceived as having anything to do with ethnobotany.

A few years ago, when cattle mutilations were plaguing northern New Mexico, a mysterious substance found near one mutilated carcass was presented to one of the authors for identification. The substance consisted of a frothy liquid in which were suspended the remains of apples, pears, Russian olives, and evening-primrose flowers. The appearance of the evening-primrose flowers brought to mind an Indian story.

EVENING-PRIMROSE pg. 239

In this particular fable all the animals were sitting in a circle discussing what gift each one brought to enhance the world. When it was coyote's turn, he was unable to think of anything he was good for. Then, in a moment of inspiration, he said, "I can make flowers," whereupon he regurgitated the evening-primrose flowers he had eaten earlier just to fill his empty stomach. His effort was rebuffed, and he was cast out of the circle of animals, and there he has remained throughout centuries of "coyote" stories. Although we were familiar with coyote's omnivorous diet, the story about the evening-primrose was a revelation. Yes, you also have guessed the source of the "mysterious" substance in this coyote's tale.

Ethnobotany comes in many guises, and its contribution to the well-being of people has not been trivial. Ethnobotany is concerned with the chemical and nutritional value of native plants for cultural groups, be they contemporary or prehistoric. In some parts of the United States during the early 1900s, a diet of nearly all yellow cornmeal resulted in an epidemic of pellagra, a disease caused by insufficient niacin. Although the Hopi diet has consisted mostly of corn (maize), they have not suffered from pellagra because they consume blue corn, which is much higher in niacin than regular corn. The Hopi's relative good health also may be due to their use of a wood ash in processing corn, for wood ash is known to enhance the niacin content of cornmeal. Fourwing saltbush, a woody shrub often used prehistorically as fuel, has been identified as the plant that Hopi traditionally burn for the ash, which they then eat with

FOURWING SALTBUSH pg. 152

or use in the preparation of corn. It is interesting to note that the use of wet wood ash or another alkaline substance in the preparation of corn for human consumption improves the availability of niacin and other amino acids and thus plays an important role in preventing protein deficiency.

The incidence of diabetes is especially high in the Western American Indian population. Presently, and due in considerable part to the interest of ethnobotanists such as Gary Paul Nabhan, an effort is being made to encourage the use of native plant foods, which are high in bulk and substances that stabilize blood-sugar levels and, therefore, are ideal for diabetics. Indeed, they are good for all of us.

Archaeobotany is the study of plant parts found in a setting related to people and their culture. In our area, the settings are typically prehistoric ruins, storage caches, cave dwellings, or rock shelters. Retrieval of charred seeds, fruit, and other plant remains from these places is most successful when the technique of flotation is employed. In this method, a prescribed amount of dirt or debris from a carefully selected feature, such as a hearth or midden, is poured into water. Material that floats to the surface is skimmed off and dried, and the remaining mixture is poured through a series of stacked, size-graded sieves. Items thus collected are then dried, placed in envelopes, and labeled with their provenience (that is, exactly where and at what level they came from in the excavation). Without this contextual information, the samples lose much of their capacity to inform us about past plant uses.

Fine paint brushes and needles are used to separate the organic remains from the other material in the dry sample. Separated materials are then examined using a binocular microscope with a power of magnification from ten to fifty times the object's size. Frequently, the items being examined are charred. As it happens, charred plant parts are much more likely to be prehistoric than uncharred specimens. In open sites, such as archaic living areas in sand dunes, hearth stones and bits of charred plant remains and pollen may be all that is left to be excavated. After examining some thirty-five thousand plant remains from a large Four Corners ruin, archaeobotanists concluded that the greater bulk of plant material had been lost to foraging insects and rodents. Nevertheless, archaeobotany can give a very accurate account of some of the plants that were important to ancient people.

When an ethnobotanist works with a specimen, he or she must refer to a comparative reference collection. The collection might be in the form of preserved tree-ring cores, an herbarium of pressed plants, or on microscope slides featuring known pollens. Drawers filled with identified modern seeds, fibers, wood, and other diagnostic parts of plants or even collections of charcoal, prehistoric corncobs, animal scats, coprolites, and insects are items an ethnobotanist uses in his or her work.

It is helpful to be able to identify a plant from the ethnic area of study during any period of its life cycle, that is, from seed to seedling, flower to fruit, and fruit to seed. Since these stages are dependent upon local climate, this study of phenology provides data on the seasonal resources for the contemporary as well as prehistoric peoples. Further, clues will already be in place as to the identity of the plant, and the antiquity of its use is revealed when one is in the field with a native colleague and he points out a plant and explains how it was used by his immediate and distant ancestors.

It is also important to know what pests, such as grasshoppers and weevils, ancient people had to contend with both on their crops and in their storage bins. We know squash bugs are nearly as old as squash, and that cotton weevils are as old as cotton. Creatures as enduring as these are not likely to be eliminated soon. In fact, they have been immortalized on prehistoric pots and on rock surfaces. Archaeologists also like to know what pests they have to contend with that might have eaten the evidence.

Small seeds, insects, termite pellets, and other minute organic remains that one can see with the naked eye (but not necessarily well enough to recognize them) or by using a relatively low-power microscope are euphemistically called "macrofossils." In contrast, desiccated plant remains that are so small that they require for examination a very high-power microscope are called *microfossils*, and they are measured in microns, which measure one millionth of a meter. (The head of a pin is about 100 microns in diameter.) Microfossils include such minutiae as pollen grains, pinworms, and spiny-headed worms, as well as *phytoliths*, the distinctive, silicon-filled molds of dead plant cells. All of the above have been extracted from prehistoric desiccated human feces.

People pellets (a term coined by an archaeobotanist of some delicacy), better known as coprolites or desiccated human feces, are prepared and studied much the same way as macrofossils and microfossils are. Those from Danger Cave in Utah revealed that lice have been associated with people in the Southwest for at least three thousand years. Pinworms, found in so many of the ancient human scats from Mesa Verde, suggest that the entire population was probably infected. These human scourges are definitely pre-Columbian.

Malnutrition and a resultant weakened human body made early people especially vulnerable to disease. One major contributor to the spread of contagious disease must have been the lack of sanitation. Archaeologists are amazed at the number of human coprolites found in or within proximity to prehistoric living quarters.

Evidence of malnutrition is often apparent in the bones of human skeletons. Conversely, no such evidence mars the skeleton of a well-nourished individual. On Black Mesa in northeastern Arizona, prehistoric skeletal remains indicated that nearly everyone, with the exception of high-status males in special burials, had as a child a type of cranial osteoporosis caused by dietary deficiency. Skeletal remains indicate that by adulthood the diet of males improved so much that they were able to overcome the disease, whereas adult women remained afflicted. Children were the most consistently stressed, and every child suffered from more than one disease caused by a poor or insufficient diet or ill health. What we can infer from existing evidence is that females and children received less nourishing food than males, with high-status males receiving the highest amount (Gumerman 1984). Perhaps one reason for this discrepancy is that men and older boys did the hunting and thus were able to eat smaller game they caught when out on expeditions while the women and children ate a virtually vegetarian diet.

Vegetables contain vitamins and minerals and the leaves of some goosefoots even contain a fair amount of protein, while amaranth leaves can be high in calcium and iron. If they are eaten with a mostly starchy food like corn, the nutrition of the meal is considerably improved. In terms of meeting their nutritional needs, the early spring months were a most difficult time for ancient people because most of the previous year's food supply was depleted and the new year's protein-rich plant foods of seeds and nuts were not yet available.

Pollen, the semen of the flowering plant world, is minutely proportioned and magnificently durable. The study of pollen is called *palynology*. Pollen from flowering plants may be found in soil strata at archaeological excavation sites, in the scrapings of a bowl left near a hearth, in coprolites, and in many other contexts. Pollen is nearly indestructible, and like seeds and other remains, it provides cultural information when it is found in association with food items, food processing tools, vessels, ceremonial objects, special activity areas, or anything else used by humans.

Plants are pollinated by the accidental action of a breeze, insects foraging in blossoms, and even water drops that fall from one flower to another. Like macrofossils, pollen can indicate what plants were growing in close proximity to an ancient pueblo or community, what weedy or semicultivated plants were allowed to grow in gardens, and what plants were probably eaten. Pollen may suggest an interpretation of the vegetation and ecozone in which the prehistoric site was situated. Airborne tree pollen can, in a general way, indicate what trees and other plant resources were perhaps available at a greater distance. Ancient pollen samples are easily contaminated by modern pollen and must be collected with the most stringent protocols.

As shown by the archaeobotanical record, the close correspondence between prehistoric and modern taxa at many prehistoric sites in the Four Corners suggests that, except for effects brought about by man, livestock, and short-term climate fluctuations, the differences between local plant communities of today and those of two thousand years ago are minor.

At the Mesa Verde complex, pollen data from stratigraphic columns indicate that a near-climax forest existed when the region was first occupied. Coprolites from a later period in the ruin show times marked by less forest pollen and a concomitant rise in pollen from garden weeds such as amaranth, goosefoot, and beeweed, and especially from the cultigen corn. Still later, corn pollen decreases along with that of garden weeds, while pollens from sagebrush, cactus, ricegrass, and other wild plants increase. Following the final abandonment of the area, the rise in pine pollen is so obvious that it has been linked to natural reforestation.

Dendrochronology, the study of tree rings, provides the best method for dating southwestern archaeological ruins. Briefly, a core or cross section of a tree is extracted and examined with each ring width being measured. A single growth ring formed during the growing season usually equals one year. Rings differ in color, dark being wood produced at the end of the growing season and light being spring or summer wood. Wider rings indicate that more water was available to the tree that year and narrow rings indicate limited water availability. Correlating a series of rings with other trees of known age has resulted in a multicentury tree-ring dating record for the Four Corners. When presented with a sufficient cross section of tree wood from prehistoric structures, dendrochronologists can determine in what year the tree was cut, the relative amount of moisture that particular tree received in different years, and, by inference, the periods of adequate precipitation and years of drought.

Some conifers are also sensitive to temperature, and the yearly records of their rings may also infer the relative coldness or warmth of the prehistoric seasons. Tree rings thus represent both a chronological record and indications of local climatic conditions. The climate was certainly critical for prehistoric agriculturalists just as it is today for modern farmers in the Four Corners area.

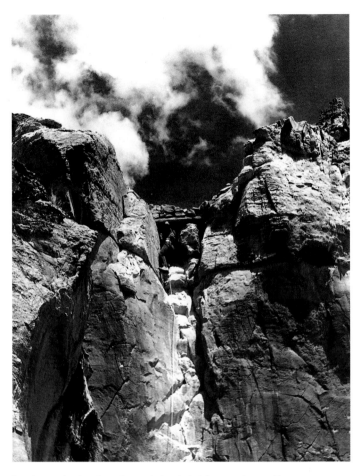

Roped researcher from Crow Canyon Archaeological Center coring wood beams at Ancestral Puebloan site.

The methods and techniques of archaeobotanical discovery are constantly evolving. Among the more recent techniques of inquiry is the study of phytoliths, which are silicon-filled dead plant cells. The cells act as molds that give their shape to the silicon as it enters into a solution and then hardens. It has been discovered that certain related groups of plants have distinctively shaped phytoliths: some are dumbbell-shaped, others

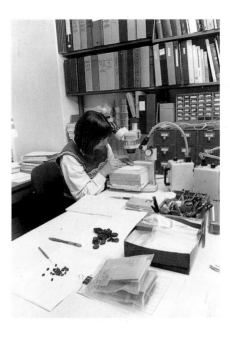

Ethnobotanist Mollie Toll at work in her lab.

cross-shaped, etc. Phytoliths, like pollen, require complicated and potentially hazardous extraction by means of chemicals. Because of the remarkable state of preservation of perishable plant materials in the dry Southwest, archaeobotanists often use phytoliths only when seeds, fruits, wood, and even pollen are disintegrated, distorted, degraded beyond recognition, or unavailable.

Restrictions have been placed upon the study of the corporeal remains of prehistoric people by their descendants. Some of the new techniques, such as DNA studies on skeletons, as well as some of the old ones, such as examining stomach contents, are considered intrusive and offensive by many native people. Today prehistoric human remains exhumed accidentally or during archaeological excavations are regularly reburied nearby or returned to their nearest living relatives for suitable reburial. The Hopi, for example, are called upon to help with reburial of ancient ancestor remains that are unearthed on the Ute Mountain Ute Reservation or at Mesa Verde National Park. Some Indian tribes are finding that archaeologists and ethnologists can be helpful in verifying their ancestors, their ancestral lands, and their sacred landforms.

Plant DNA remains readily available, and since its extraction is an acceptable practice, it is a potentially powerful tool in the study of plant and human coevolution. The journeys of domesticated, semidomesticated, and wild plants such as wolf-berry (*Lycium* spp.) and tobacco (*Nicotiana* spp.) seem to have been influenced by prehistoric human activity, and they may one day be mapped (Karen Adams, personal communication, 1996). In the process, a plant's genotypic changes may be related to specific groups of people. Such changes might reflect the choices the ancient ancestors made in selecting attributes for domesticated and semidomesticated plants. Drought resistance and larger, more rapidly developing fruit are two characteristics preferred by southwestern farming people. Indian gardeners are still selecting for the characteristics they prefer in vegetables and grains and saving the seed. Some Hopi families do not allow seed corn out of the house except to be blessed or planted. All other corn from their fields is cooked before it is dried, thereby rendering the grain useless for propagation. In many cases, the results of this care are rare heirloom seeds.

WOLFBERRY
pg. 180

A few organizations such as Native Seeds/SEARCH are attempting to preserve seed of these oldest varieties and grow them out within a five-year period. After five years the ability of a seed to germinate declines precipitously. All seed banks are having difficulty complying with this necessary but restricted timetable. Ethnobotanists are collecting the germ plasm, or seeds, but there are too few farmers and not enough separate small plots of land available to grow out hundreds of cultivated varieties and keep them from cross-pollinating.

Several renowned ethnobiological laboratories focus their study on the Southwest. One special study center in the heart of the Four Corners, Crow Canyon Archaeological Center near Cortez, Colorado, is not only a research institution but also, through the use of hands-on techniques, a center for the education of students, teachers, and the public. Through these efforts they train enthusiastic and competent future archaeobotanists and archaeologists.

Karen Adams, director of the Environmental Archaeology Program at Crow Canyon, is devising ingenious, small studies to provide data and further the interpretation of the faunal and floral remains at archaeological sites in the Four Corners region. One experiment utilized known varieties of indigenous southwestern corn. The mature corn ears, including kernels and cobs, were photographed, weighed, and measured. Then the cobs were placed in a very hot fire that simulated an ancient hearth in which leftover cobs were used as fuel. Before-and-after pictures showed that the charred maize shrank up to two-thirds of its overall dimensions, looking for all the world like some of the "primitive" tiny cobs recovered from many prehistoric sites.

Suggested Reading

Balick, Michael J. and Paul Alan Cox
1996   *Plants, People, and Culture: The Science of Ethnobotany.* Scientific American Library, New York.

Bohrer, Vorsila L.
1986   Guideposts in Ethnobotany. *Journal of Ethnobiology* 6(1):27–43.

Ford Richard I.
1978   *The Nature and Status of Ethnobotany.* Anthropological Papers no. 67. University of Michigan, Museum of Anthropology, Ann Arbor.

Gumerman, George J.
1984   *A View from Black Mesa: The Changing Face of Archaeology.* University of Arizona Press, Tucson and London.

Martin, Gary J.
1995   *Ethnobotany.* Chapman and Hall, London.

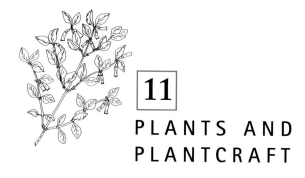

11

PLANTS AND PLANTCRAFT

T HE FOUR CORNERS REGION of Colorado, Utah,
Arizona, and New Mexico lies roughly within
one hundred miles of the actual intersection of
the four states as covered in this book. It is a land of enormous
natural and human diversity. This country encompasses a nine-
thousand-foot range in elevation, from around four thousand
feet along the San Juan River before it empties into the
Colorado, to more than thirteen thousand feet in the La Plata
Mountains just north and east of Mesa Verde.

Roughly two thousand different species of flowering plants
are native to the area. More than a quarter of these wild plants
are known to have been used in one way or another by the prehistoric Indians or the Hopi, Navajo, Ute, and Jicarilla Apache.
More than sixty of them are covered in the plant descriptions
that follow—plants that are considered to be both important to
native peoples and that are readily seen in the wild today, especially along the roads and trails of the five featured parks.

The plants are grouped by growth form—trees, shrubs,
grasses, and herbaceous plants—then arranged by plant family

in phylogenetic order, that is, those most closely related, which is the sequence found in most technical plant manuals. Each description includes common and scientific names for the species or group of species. Throughout the text, sp. refers to singular species; spp. refers to plural species.

The principal distinguishing characteristics are described for each plant, accompanied by line drawings and a color photograph emphasizing those features. Diagramatic drawings of seeds that come from edible fruit, or that might be found in an archaeological context, accompany the plant drawings. The actual size range of the seeds is depicted by the cluster near the enlarged rendering. In addition, we provide information about a particular species's habitat, its flowering season, and where it might be found in the parks covered in this book.

Some of the plants will need to be in flower for positive identification. Fortunately, the flowering period for most extends over many weeks and coincides with the season you are likely to be visiting the parks.

In a few cases, as with the joint-firs (*Ephedra* spp.), we treat the genus as a single entity rather than differentiating several species that are difficult to tell apart without using a magnifying glass and a technical plant identification key. Typically, most Indian users of such closely related plants look upon them as a single group, and so do we.

We direct you to five different parks in the National Park System where you are likely to find the profiled plants. Within each of these archaeological parks, we indicate the most popular roads, trails, or campgrounds for plant searches. Each park has a visitor center that provides maps and informational materials about the trails and particular points of interest. A brief description of the five featured parks follows, along with addresses for obtaining more information.

Chaco Culture National Historical Park is the place where Ancestral Puebloan architecture reached a zenith during a two-hundred-year period starting in the early A.D. 900s. In this northwestern New Mexico park that lies southeast of Farmington you can see well-interpreted ruins, learn about the

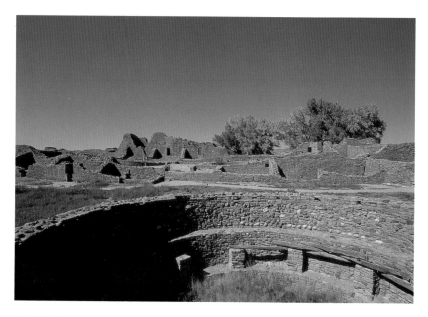

Aztec Ruins National Monument.

early Chacoans at the modern park museum, and take a ranger-conducted walk along one of many trails. Many of the useful plants described in this book will be seen from the canyon-bottom loop road, the trail to Pueblo Alto, or at the Gallo Campground. Plants and their prehistoric uses often are topics at ranger-conducted talks. Plan to spend at least a day. Open daily, but unpaved roads are difficult to negotiate during inclement weather. There is no lodging, gasoline, or auto repair service at the park; modest visitor-use fee. National Park Service, Star Route 4, Box 6500, Bloomfield, New Mexico 87413.

Aztec Ruins National Monument Sometime during the early 1100s, people with ties to Chaco built a pueblo-style village along the Animas River where it flows out onto the plains from the mountainous country to the north. Today a self-guiding trail leads you through the main ruins of this ancient settlement that was once connected by a road system to Chaco. Along this trail and at the adjacent picnic area you will encounter several of the useful plants mentioned in this book. The Park Service visitor center is on the outskirts of the city of Aztec. Open daily; modest visitor-use fee. National Park Service, P. O. Box 640, Aztec, New Mexico 87410.

Mesa Verde National Park was established in 1906 and is the most well-known and best-developed archaeological park in the country. Located in southwestern Colorado between Durango and Cortez, Mesa Verde preserves thousands of prehistoric ruins spanning nearly eight hundred years of the Ancestral Puebloan era. Self-guiding trails incorporate wild plants and their ancient uses into the interpretive story; museum exhibits and ranger-guided walks and talks also are informative. Although most of the backcountry ruins are off-limits, many of the best examples are accessible to the public. Following the 5,000-acre fire of 1996, Mesa Verde offers an extra bonus. Visitors can learn about the mostly positive effects of natural fire and see for themselves how the park is renewed through nature's grand display of vegetational change.

Mesa Verde is home to the greatest number of plants discussed in this book. The main road leading to Park Headquarters, the one-way interpretive loop drives on Chapin Mesa, the trail to Spruce Tree House, and the huge Morefield Campground are excellent places to see these plants. Plan to spend at least a full day here. Open daily, but some facilities are closed in winter; entrance fee for vehicles. National Park Service, Mesa Verde National Park, P. O. Box 8, Colorado 81330-0008.

Hovenweep National Monument is remarkable for its series of spectacular towers and other stone structures built by Ancestral Puebloans, some of whom may have been related to those living at Mesa Verde. Several gravel roads lead to this out-of-the-way park on Utah's eastern boundary due west of Cortez, Colorado. The self-guiding Square Tower Loop Trail provides a good introduction to Hovenweep and is a great short

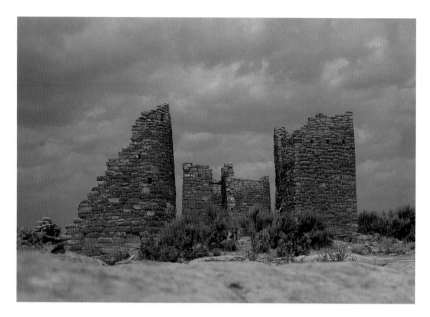

Hovenweep Castle, Hovenweep National Monument.

hike for seeing a variety of useful plants. Open daily; modest visitor-use fee. The park is administered as a unit of Mesa Verde. National Park Service, McElmo Route, Cortez, Colorado 81321.

Canyon de Chelly National Monument combines awesome Southwest canyon scenery with Ancestral Puebloan ruins and more recent Navajo Indian habitations and agricultural fields. Paved roads lead to spectacular overlooks along the rims of the two major canyons. A museum and visitor center are located just east of Chinle, Arizona, as are a wide range of facilities, including a public campground. The park is within the Navajo Indian Reservation; open-air vehicle tours into the canyon are provided for a fee by Navajo guides. Many of the most useful wild plants will be seen along South and North Rim drives and by the short, improved trails to canyon overlooks. Contact the superintendent at Box 588, Chinle, Arizona 86503 for information and to book tours into the canyon.

Remember that the rules of all these parks (as well as those sites described in chapter 12, "Other Places to Visit,") prohibit the disturbance of natural or cultural features. When it comes to the wild plants we describe here or to any other plants in the parks, never pick them: "Leave nothing but footprints; take nothing but pictures."

The descriptions of plant uses include both prehistoric and, if known, recent associations. All references to ancient and historic plant uses in this book come from original sources including published materials, our own observations, and discussions with various contemporary authorities and native people from the Four Corners region.

The Concept of Ecozones

In the plant descriptions that follow, we often refer to the vegetative community, or ecozone, where that particular species is most likely to be found. Ecozones are defined by the dominant plants, usually one or more tree species, that characterize the pattern of vegetation in a given area.

Each zone is a reflection of the local climate, mainly the annual precipitation coupled with the average temperature, which, in turn, influences how much moisture is available for plant growth. The chart shown here depicts how annual precipitation increases with elevation, resulting in a gradient of increasing annual moisture from the lowest basins to the summits of the highest mountain ranges in the Four Corners region.

The effect of exposure (determined by the direction a slope faces) creates an additional influence on available moisture. South-facing slopes benefit from more direct sunlight and have higher daily temperatures throughout the year whereas colder, north-facing slopes retain soil moisture for a longer period. The

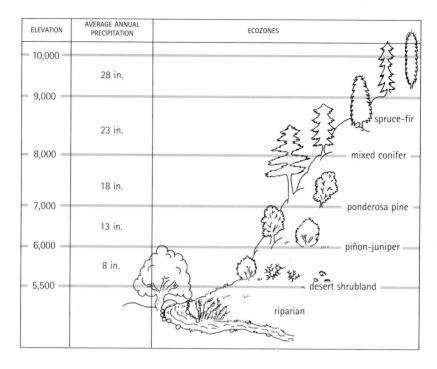

ELEVATION	AVERAGE ANNUAL PRECIPITATION	ECOZONES
10,000	28 in.	spruce-fir
9,000		
8,000	23 in.	mixed conifer
7,000	18 in.	ponderosa pine
6,000	13 in.	piñon-juniper
5,500	8 in.	desert shrubland / riparian

result is that a given ecozone occurring on the north side of a mountain will be found at a considerably higher elevation—as much as one thousand feet higher—on the south side.

All the species mentioned in the plant profiles live in one of four ecozones: desert shrubland, piñon-juniper, ponderosa pine, or mixed conifer. Most of the useful plants are concentrated in the two lowest zones. While another ecozone, spruce-fir, exists in the Four Corners, it occurs near the summits of the higher mountain ranges, beyond where native people regularly traveled and collected. Flowing streams, ponds, or drainages with abundant subsurface moisture provide a specialized environment that can support water-requiring plants such as cottonwood, willow, or common reed. In these situations, in places such as alongside the San Juan River, Chaco Wash, or the bottom of Canyon de Chelly, a distinctive riparian vegetative community takes over.

The Plants

PIÑON PINE

Pine family
(*Pinus edulis*)

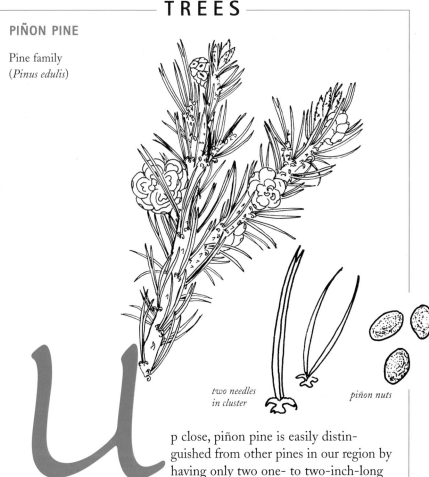

*two needles
in cluster*

piñon nuts

U p close, piñon pine is easily distinguished from other pines in our region by
having only two one- to two-inch-long
needles in each bundle and, from a distance, by its rounded crown and
irregular shape. They may be the slowest growing of all pines, and
their age at maturity ranges from seventy-five to two hundred years,
with the oldest occasionally reaching four hundred years.

Piñon-juniper evergreen woodlands dominate mesas and lower
mountain slopes in the Four Corners region. The range for piñon pine
extends a bit higher than for Utah juniper, so at the upper end of the
piñon-juniper, or p-j, zone, the woodland is almost pure piñon, as on
the higher mesa tops at Mesa Verde. Along with junipers, piñons are
the most common trees in the parks covered here except for Chaco,
where they are rarely encountered today.

Few trees produce bountiful seed crops every year, and the piñon is no exception. Initial cone formation is dependent upon moisture in late winter or early spring; once formed, the cones and nuts do not mature until eighteen months later. Nuts are fully developed and ready for gathering in late August, but a bumper crop can be expected only once every six years.

For Archaic Indians, Ancestral Puebloans, and historic tribes living in this region in the early days, piñon pine was surely the tree of life. Cracked nutshells are found at virtually all Ancestral Puebloan sites. At Chaco, however, shell remains were far fewer than would have been predicted despite the fact that these pines were common around the canyon during the earlier time of habitation. The reason for this is not known (Mollie S. Toll, personal communication, 1996).

The Hopi, Navajo, Ute, and Jicarilla Apache all ate wild piñon nuts, and most do today. In earlier times the cones may have been green when picked and stored, protecting the nuts from rodents. In winter the cones were put on hot coals that forced them to spring open.

Of course, roasted or raw piñon nuts are delicious by anyone's standards, but more important is their caloric value: piñon nuts contain more than three thousand calories per pound. They also contain the twenty amino acids that make up complete protein, and the value of the nut's protein on a per-pound basis is comparable to that of steak. Of the nine amino acids essential to human growth, seven are more concentrated in these nuts than in corn. Along with peppergrass greens and seeds, piñon nuts are an excellent source of potassium.

Several tribes applied pitch, which oozes out of the tree trunk and collects on the bark, to cuts and sores to protect them from exposure to air. Navajo burned this resin to create fumes to cure a head cold. Navajo household remedies included preparing an extract made from pine and juniper needles to treat headaches, coughs, and fevers. Earaches were treated by fumigation with pulverized dry buds.

Piñon pitch, usually boiled down, had many practical uses as an adhesive and sealer. It was used by the Hopi to waterproof and repair pottery, by the Navajo to cement turquoise stones into silverwork, and by the Ute to repair sandals. Traditional water jugs woven from branches of willow or threeleaf sumac are sealed on the inside and outside with melted piñon gum. With their shiny appearance these

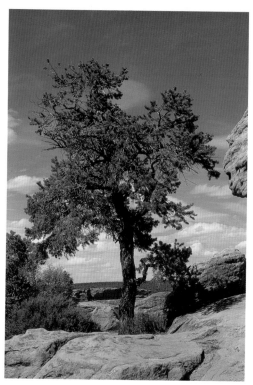
Piñon pine

containers are easily identified among other baskets displayed at trading posts.

Ute Mountain Utes smoked hides for tepees and various bags over a piñon wood fire to produce a light yellow tint. Navajo Indians mix the pitch with a boiled extract of threeleaf sumac leaves and yellow ocher to make a black dye for wool.

Before the day of Wrigley's, many a Four Corners resident chewed on piñon pitch for the simple pleasure of it.

UTAH JUNIPER

Cypress family
(*Juniperus osteosperma*)

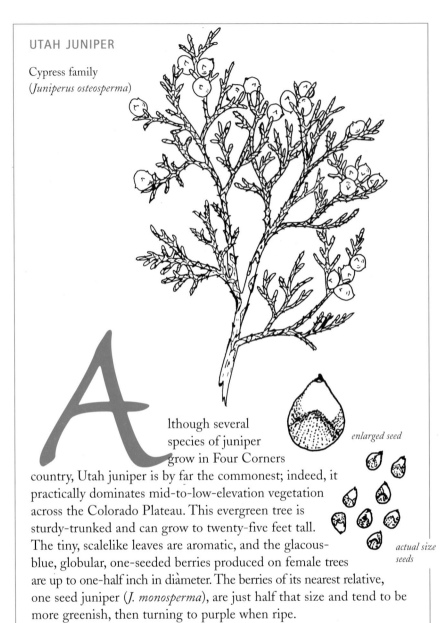

enlarged seed

actual size seeds

Although several species of juniper grow in Four Corners country, Utah juniper is by far the commonest; indeed, it practically dominates mid-to-low-elevation vegetation across the Colorado Plateau. This evergreen tree is sturdy-trunked and can grow to twenty-five feet tall. The tiny, scalelike leaves are aromatic, and the glacous-blue, globular, one-seeded berries produced on female trees are up to one-half inch in diameter. The berries of its nearest relative, one seed juniper (*J. monosperma*), are just half that size and tend to be more greenish, then turning to purple when ripe.

Utah juniper, usually mixed with piñon pine, defines the mesa-top woodlands at Mesa Verde and Canyon de Chelly and is the major tree at Hovenweep as well. At Chaco the few evergreen trees seen along the trail to Pueblo Alto are one-seed junipers. Rocky Mountain

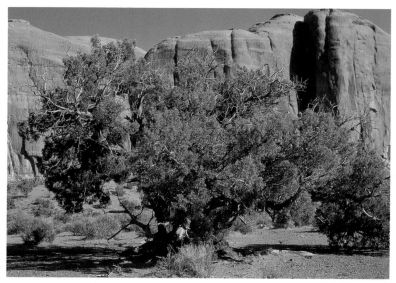

Utah juniper

juniper (*J. scopulorum*), with its more delicate, drooping branches, grows along the trail to Spruce Tree House at Mesa Verde, as does the Utah juniper. Westerners frequently refer to junipers as "cedars" even though they are not at all like the true cedars of the genus *Cedrus*, which are native to the Old World.

Throughout the Southwest, junipers have enjoyed a greater variety of Native American uses than any other group of wild plants. Analyzed coprolites from Chaco, Mesa Verde, and other Ancestral Puebloan sites confirm that juniper berries were regularly eaten. Although the berries of Utah juniper are rather dry and mealy, they make up for it in their generous size. All native peoples living around the Four Corners have relied on juniper berries for food at one time or another, especially during famine. The Hopi used to like to eat the berries with their piki bread, and the Navajo use water laced with ashes from burned juniper branches to make blue cornbread.

Medicinal applications for Utah juniper are legion. This is especially true for the Navajo, for whom it is a revered plant. Sweathouses are made with juniper wood, and juniper bark covers their floors. Various infusions of juniper twigs and leaves, sometimes mixed

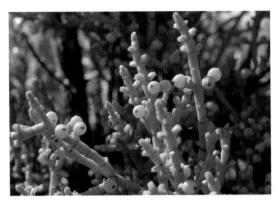

Juniper mistletoe

with other plants, are used by the Navajo to treat colds, headaches, stomachaches, nausea, acne, and spider bites.

Hopi and almost all other Pueblo women have a tradition of drinking juniper-sprig tea during labor or immediately after a child is born. An extract of juniper and sagebrush leaves has long been used to treat indigestion by the Hopi; thus, it is not surprising that this mixture has been observed in coprolites from Ancestral Puebloan sites, suggesting that these plants were used in prehistoric medicines.

At many prehistoric villages juniper was not as widely used in construction as other trees. Only 4 percent of the wood beams at Pueblo Bonito in Chaco Canyon were of juniper, but juniper bark was favored by the Ute for covering their wickiups, which often were built of juniper branches and poles. However, Ute Indians avoided burning juniper in the central wickiup fire pit because "it might pop and set the shelter on fire" (Smith 1974). In less flammable structures, juniper fuelwood is preferred for heating hogans or other homes because it burns with a hot flame and little smoke.

Juniper is a Navajo dye plant for wool. A boiled liquid of twigs, leaves, and berries produces yellow to orange shades of tan. A mordant to fix other Navajo dyes is derived from juniper leaf ashes, which is traditionally used with mountain-mahogany root bark ashes to dye buckskin moccasins red. The Hopi don't use juniper to create dyes, but both groups string the seeds into necklaces that one sees for sale throughout the region.

Juniper bark is easily stripped in long, loose strands from mature trees, and it was used by Ancestral Puebloans to manufacture cordage, legging insulation, roofing material, and even toilet paper. At Aztec Ruins, juniper bark was wrapped with yucca to fashion prehistoric pot rests.

At one time the Ute used juniper bark in their cordage. More recently they have made hunting bows from juniper wood. Navajo also crafted juniper bows as well as hoops for a baby's cradle, but unlike many Puebloans, they avoided using juniper bark as a cradle matting. According to Navajos, juniper bark gives babies a rash, thus these people prefer to use shreddy cliffrose bark for cradle matting.

Even the profuse, yellow-green mistletoe (*Phoradendron juniperinum*) that often clings tenaciously to juniper branches (but does not really harm the tree) was used among the Navajo. The globular, translucent berries of juniper mistletoe were once eaten fresh, although that's no longer the case today. A boiled mixture of juniper and piñon sprigs plus mistletoe is made into a lotion used to treat ant and other insect bites.

COYOTE WILLOW

Willow family
(*Salix exigua*)

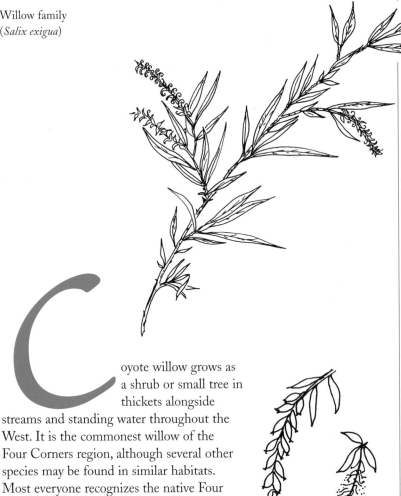

Coyote willow grows as a shrub or small tree in thickets alongside streams and standing water throughout the West. It is the commonest willow of the Four Corners region, although several other species may be found in similar habitats. Most everyone recognizes the native Four Corners willows from their thin, flexible branches, narrow leaves, and the fluffy, spike-shaped female flower clusters called catkins that appear in spring.

female catkin

male catkin

Willows grow along the flowing or surface-dry streambeds in the parks discussed in this book; however, due to lowered water tables, they are not as common today along Chaco Wash as they probably once were.

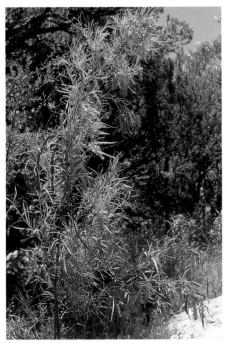
Coyote Willow

Ancestral Puebloans found endless uses for willow when it was available to them. In Canyon de Chelly the wood was used for textile loom anchors, for rods to control the weaving rhythm, and for finishing needles. Bows, arrow points, pot rests, scrapers, and cradle parts all were crafted from willow. In later times Navajo made weaving sticks and arrow shafts from willow along with other straight-grained woods, and Ute Indians made snowshoe frames from dried willow branches. Perhaps the most distinctive characteristic of a Ute cradleboard is the willowwork basketry covering that provided shade for the baby (Pettit 1990).

Matting was another early product made from willow. In 1919 Earl Morris described such a mat uncovered during the excavation of Aztec Ruins: "It was 2 feet long by 2 feet 7 inches wide, and consisted of sixty-eight willows strung on ten yucca cords. One side of the willows had been flattened so as to give the mat a flat instead of a transversely ribbed surface. On the back of the mat the bark had not been removed from the willows" (Morris 1919).

In Ancestral Puebloan times, willow, along with threeleaf sumac, was the material of choice for manufacturing Native American baskets. Willow wands tend to be a little stouter than those of threeleaf sumac and thus often were used to produce courser basketry. Jicarilla Apache basketmaker Lydia Pesata told us that willow is harder to dye than sumac because the bark is slicker and the dye doesn't take as well. Lydia collects willow just after spring when the bark is not too slick.

Coyote willow grows most plentifully in the northwest quadrant of the Four Corners Area where the climate is wetter. Thus, at one time it was preferred by the Ute Mountain Ute for building usually near streams the domed houses they occupied in summer.

Ute Indians used to concoct a green dye for coloring buckskin by soaking willow leaves in hot water and then boiling the mixture to concentrate the pigment. Willow roots also have been used by others to manufacture a rose-tan dye.

Willow leaves are among a large number of plant parts that Navajo healers prescribe as ceremonial emetics for their patients. Most Indians living in the Southwest are also familiar with medicinal teas brewed from willow bark used to treat upset stomachs, headaches, fevers, and inflammation. The healing property is salicylic acid, the basic ingredient of aspirin, and it is found in all willow bark and roots.

More than 2,400 years ago the Greeks learned to use extracts of several native willows to treat pain, gout, and other illnesses. In more recent times, in 1839, salicylic acid was isolated from wild plants and manufactured synthetically. Early salicylic acid–based products had unpleasant side effects. Sixty years later the Bayer Company developed a derivative of salicylic acid, called it aspirin, and the rest is history.

FREMONT COTTONWOOD

Willow family
(*Populus fremontii*)

ASPEN

(*Populus tremuloides*)

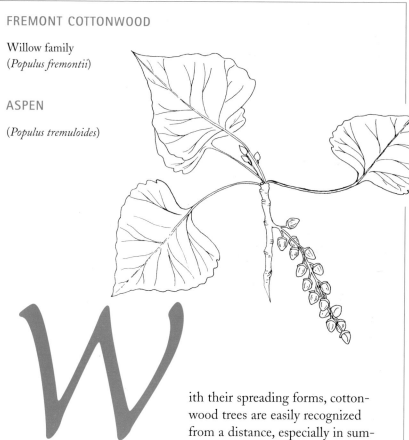

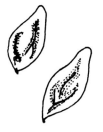

With their spreading forms, cottonwood trees are easily recognized from a distance, especially in summer when the leaves are bright green. The commonest species growing in broad valleys and along watercourses in our region is the Fremont cottonwood. It has deltoid leaves that turn golden in autumn and fall before the first snow flies. Quaking aspen grows on open slopes above 6,500 feet elevation here (but down to sea level in the northeast Atlantic states), often invading after a wildfire has cleared off the conifers. Greenish to white bark and nearly round shimmering leaves give this tree away. Aspen, too, turns to a brilliant gold in fall.

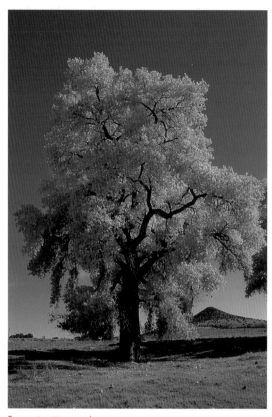
Fremont cottonwood

Cottonwoods dominate the riparian environment at Chaco, Aztec Ruins, and Canyon de Chelly, less so at Hovenweep. A few trees are scattered throughout the park at Mesa Verde. Both Mesa Verde and Canyon de Chelly support some small stands of aspen, but the other parks are too low for this species.

Fremont cottonwood seems to have been the tree of choice whenever a soft or light wood was needed by the Ancestral Puebloans. To date, the most complete information about how these people used wood from cottonwood comes to us from the excavation of Antelope House in Canyon de Chelly. Functional items recovered here include nineteen fire-making hearths and five drills, five scrapers, one awl, three bows, twenty miscellaneous rods, two shafts, and countless wooden discs or tablets. At Pueblo Bonito in Chaco Canyon one out of every eight roof beams was constructed from cottonwood or aspen.

In more recent times the Navajo made weaving loom frames, cradleboards, and snowshoes from cottonwood. Before matches became available, most Indian tribes in this region favored this wood for starting fires with the fire-by-friction method. The wood was used in drill spindles and hearths and it provided some of the tinder as

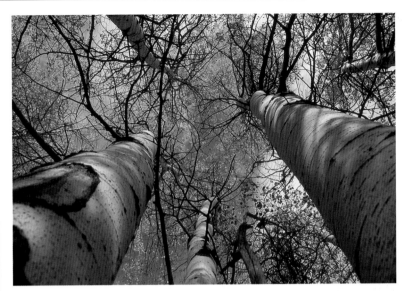
Aspen

well. Cottonwood was the preferred wood for summer fires because the flames burn bright and the fire itself is not too hot.

Early records show that the Navajo ate as an emergency ration the inner bark of aspen; Ute Indians are said to have relished the sap from these trees. Rio Grande Puebloans once ate the drooping flower clusters that appear on cottonwoods in spring before they leaf out.

The easily carved wood from both trees has been and continues to be preferred by Puebloan drum makers. After cottonwood and aspen trees die, their trunks tend to rot out in the center, making the drum makers' hollowing process easier. Cottonwood roots are *the* wood for creating Hopi and other Puebloan kachina dolls.

OAK

Oak family
(*Quercus* spp.)

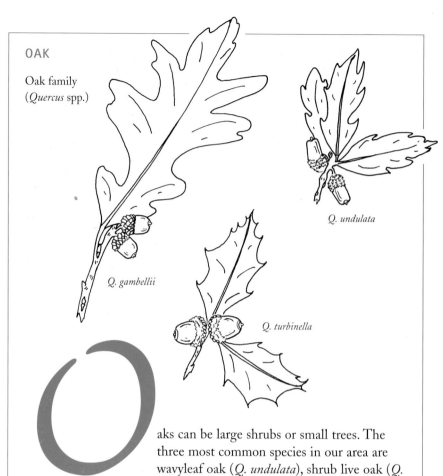

Q. undulata

Q. gambellii

Q. turbinella

Oaks can be large shrubs or small trees. The three most common species in our area are wavyleaf oak (*Q. undulata*), shrub live oak (*Q. turbinella*), and Gambel oak (*Q. gambelii*). Depending upon the species, these oaks can range from 5,000 to 8,500 feet elevation. Wavyleaf oak tends to grow between the dry environment of shrub live oak and the more moist habitat of Gambel oak. The leathery leaves of shrub live oak are one to three inches long, grayish-green on top, and fuzzy white beneath. Wavyleaf oak leaves are slightly longer and more shallowly lobed, and the only sharp point on the leaf is at its tip. Deeply lobed Gambel oak leaves, ranging from about two to seven inches long, are the largest of the southwestern oaks.

In the Four Corners, deciduous Gambel oaks are the most common of the three, and they often colonize forested mountain slopes after a fire. To see Gambel oak in mass, scan the vistas of steep slopes on the road to Mesa Verde for patches that are deep-green in summer

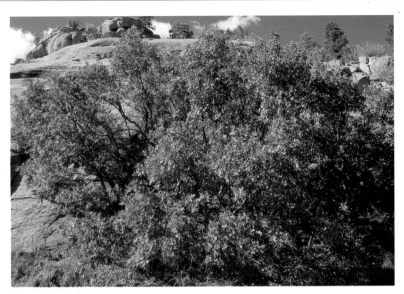
Gambel oak

or reddish-brown in the autumn. All three species occur at Canyon de Chelly.

All oaks have acorns, but unlike those of other regions, the southwestern species are sweet just as they come off the tree or shrub and need no leaching or other preparation before eating. Archaeological evidence of acorn use is scant, probably because the shells do not ordinarily endure, but some have been found in dry caves in association with very early artifacts. Acorns must have been a very important source of protein food for all early southwestern tribes. One-handed manos, thought to be used for grinding acorns, have been located by the hundreds in the southeastern part of the Four Corners region.

Roof construction at prehistoric Chaco included beams of oak. The excavation of Antelope House in Canyon de Chelly yielded numerous oak implements: bows, arrows, scoops, handles, hoes, snowshoes, and a bentwood cradle. The collection of oak implements found at Mesa Verde evinced a similar range of utility. Apparently oak was used whenever the job called for tough, pliable wood.

Rio Grande Pueblos have a long history of utilizing acorns, which were sometimes mixed with sunflowers and piñon nuts, to make nutritious mush, breads, and cakes. The wood was used to manufacture such implements as basket foundation rods, digging sticks, rabbit sticks (nonreturnable boomerangs), bows, war clubs, and medicine.

Ute Mountain Utes visited a trapper's camp in the early 1800s and brought with them acorns and other wild fruit, probably for trading (Pettit 1990). Acorns were a large and indispensable part of the Jicarilla Apache and Southern Paiute diet well into the twentieth century.

Gambel oak is a Navajo wool dye ingredient. For a tan hue, they gather the bark in fall when the strongest color is produced. Navajo also use pulverized insect galls from shrubby oaks to create a light gold or yellowish tan dye for rug wool. Some Navajo still collect acorns for food and boil them as one would beans or roast them over coals. Sometimes the acorns were dried and ground into flour. Sturdy but temporary oak-stave carrying baskets once were assembled in the field and used to carry a heavy harvest of yucca fruit. The Navajo also used oak to make bows, hoes, digging sticks, and throwing sticks used to kill rabbits and other small game. Oak is a durable, hard wood with great resistance, powerful qualities that reflect attributes of the Navajo people. This may explain why oak is used in nearly all of their ceremonies.

CHOKECHERRY

Rose family
(*Prunus virginiana*)

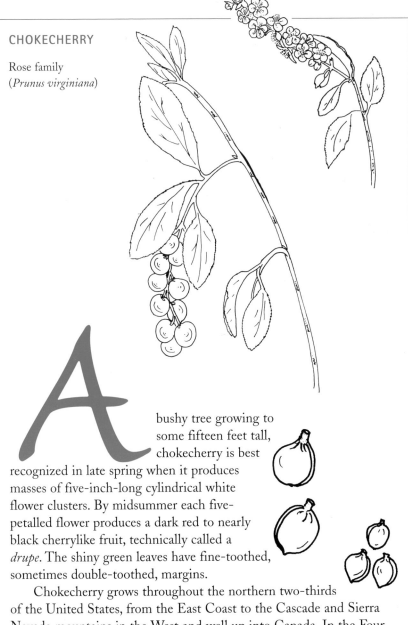

A bushy tree growing to some fifteen feet tall, chokecherry is best recognized in late spring when it produces masses of five-inch-long cylindrical white flower clusters. By midsummer each five-petalled flower produces a dark red to nearly black cherrylike fruit, technically called a *drupe*. The shiny green leaves have fine-toothed, sometimes double-toothed, margins.

Chokecherry grows throughout the northern two-thirds of the United States, from the East Coast to the Cascade and Sierra Nevada mountains in the West and well up into Canada. In the Four Corners region, where it is at the drier limit of its range, look for wild cherry trees along stream courses and on shady hillsides in the piñon-juniper and ponderosa pine ecozones. It is especially abundant along

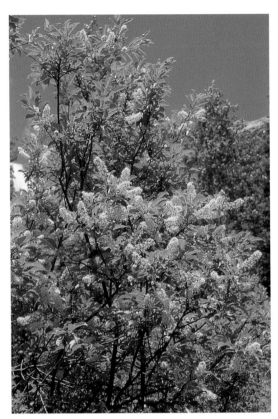
Chokecherry

the main road leading to the visitor center at Mesa Verde. Chokecherry also is fairly common at Hovenweep.

Fragments of the relatively large seeds have been identified in coprolites analyzed at Ancestral Puebloan sites throughout the Four Corners area. Although this species is considered a relatively minor component of the early diet, chokecherries must have been regularly collected and eaten by the ancients.

Chokecherries continue to be relished by native people. Jicarilla Apache once considered the fruits an indispensable staple and used to make three-inch patties from chokecherry meal. In the past, the Jicarilla would take these sweets to the northern Rio Grande pueblos during Christmas festivities. Ute Indians have regularly gathered and sun-dried the cherries, and the Navajo cook them with cornmeal. Although the fruits may be eaten raw, they are sometimes bitter. Contents of the seed stones are slightly toxic due to a fractional amount of cyanide; however, this poison is volatile and can be neutralized, for the most part, by cooking or grinding.

Because chokecherry wood is tough and flexible, it is ideal for the manufacture of bows. It was preferred by the Ute Mountain Ute for making either single- or double-backed hunting bows. Pueblo Indians living in the northern Rio Grande also made sinew-backed bows from this wood. It seems likely that Ancestral Puebloans would have used the stout, pliable limbs to make bows and other implements, but direct evidence from prehistoric sites is lacking.

Navajo weavers create a purplish-brown dye from boiled bark peeled from chokecherry roots mixed with root bark from wild plums. Jicarilla basket weaver Lydia Pesata told us that she collects the roots in early spring when the ground near her home in northern New Mexico has thawed. She then boils the root bark to create an especially deep red for dying her sumac and willow baskets. She also uses the cherries to produce a mauve color.

Chokecherry bark has been used by Pueblo Indians to concoct a cough medicine, and the dried fruit is a Life Medicine for the Navajo. Medicinal uses were widespread among Indians living in the eastern United States and were even adopted by settlers, as attested to by the following Lewis and Clark report: "When Captain Meriwether Lewis (whose mother was reported to be a "yarb [herb] doctor") was ill with abdominal cramps and fever on the upper Missouri, he took a mixture of choke cherry twigs boiled in water and was well the next day" (Vogel 1970).

JOINT-FIR

Joint-fir family
(*Ephedra* spp.)

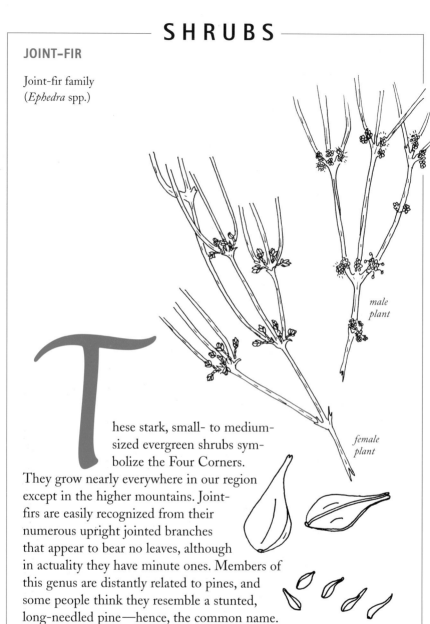

male plant

female plant

These stark, small- to medium-sized evergreen shrubs symbolize the Four Corners. They grow nearly everywhere in our region except in the higher mountains. Joint-firs are easily recognized from their numerous upright jointed branches that appear to bear no leaves, although in actuality they have minute ones. Members of this genus are distantly related to pines, and some people think they resemble a stunted, long-needled pine—hence, the common name.

Several species of *Ephedra* grow in the region, but we won't sort them out here since the differences aren't readily apparent. You can't miss seeing clumps of joint-fir at any of the parks covered in this book, with the exception of Aztec Ruins.

The fibrous stems preserve well and have been recovered from many different archaeological settings, so it is assumed that this was an important plant for making beverages in Ancestral Puebloan times. What we don't know is whether it was brewed for a pleasant-tasting tea or as a stimulating medicinal beverage.

Hopi, Ute, Southern Paiute, and Navajo have definitely used it for medicine, the latter for treating stomach pains and nasal congestion, as well as for bladder and kidney problems. Boiled roots served as a treatment for colds.

Although several early ethnologists reported that joint-fir tea was used to cure syphilis, it's more likely that it was the urinary tract disorders resulting from this disease that abated. Pseudoephedrine contained in the cells of this plant is an alkaloid that can cause constriction of blood vessels and an increase in blood pressure, leading to better filtration of urine through the kidneys.

We have been told by contemporary Indians that the tea they steep today from *Ephedra* twigs is consumed both for medicinal purposes and for pleasure. Certainly, many Anglo settlers thought of it as

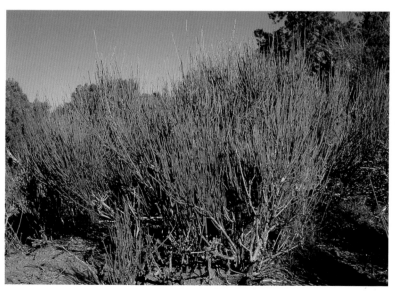

Joint-fir

a stimulating beverage, especially the Mormons, from whom comes its other popular name, Mormon tea. Because of the caffeine in regular coffee and tea, those beverages have long been prohibited by Mormon church doctrine, so Mormons sought the next best thing for an every-day pick-me-up.

Joint-fir twigs and their tiny leaves served the Navajo as a dye ingredient. Wool was boiled with the twigs mixed with raw alum to color it light tan. The Navajo occasionally used one species in place of alder bark to make a reddish dye for baskets. At Dulce, New Mexico, Lydia Pesata still uses joint-fir twigs to dye her woven Jicarilla baskets tan.

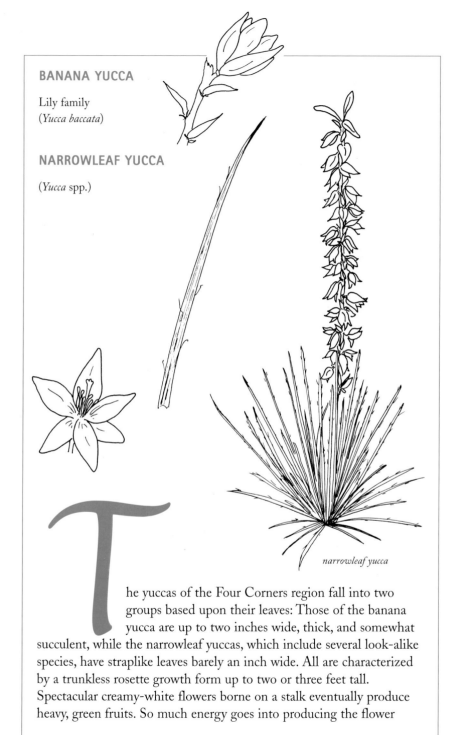

BANANA YUCCA

Lily family
(*Yucca baccata*)

NARROWLEAF YUCCA

(*Yucca* spp.)

narrowleaf yucca

The yuccas of the Four Corners region fall into two groups based upon their leaves: Those of the banana yucca are up to two inches wide, thick, and somewhat succulent, while the narrowleaf yuccas, which include several look-alike species, have straplike leaves barely an inch wide. All are characterized by a trunkless rosette growth form up to two or three feet tall. Spectacular creamy-white flowers borne on a stalk eventually produce heavy, green fruits. So much energy goes into producing the flower stalk and fruits that most yuccas bloom only once every few years. For fertilization, yuccas in the Southwest are dependent upon a night visit by a tiny, highly specialized female moth that brushes the flower's stigma with collected pollen as she enters the blossom to lay her single egg in the flower's ovary.

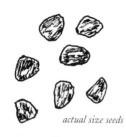

actual size seeds

Banana yucca is widespread on Chapin Mesa at Mesa Verde but less common at Aztec Ruins and Canyon de Chelly. Narrowleaf yucca is abundant at Hovenweep and Canyon de Chelly but occurs less frequently today at Chaco.

enlarged seed

With an enormous variety of uses, yuccas constitute the single most important noncultivated group of plants for prehistoric and contemporary Indians living in the Southwest. One of the basic requirements for a people progressing toward a more advanced society would have been the ability to tie one object to another; to do this, you usually need some kind of cordage. The long, tough fibers that could be extracted from yucca leaves played a fundamental role in early weaving, manufacturing, and construction, especially before cotton was imported from the South. Yucca fibers were twisted or braided into twine and rope that were used for lashing house beams, fixing ladder rungs, fashioning blankets or belts, making bowstrings and nets for fishing or trapping small game, sewing animal-skin robes, and binding together all manner of items. (See page 91 for methods of preparing yucca fibers.)

Much more recently, in an experiment during World War II, fibers from narrowleaf yucca growing in the wild were commercially extracted and made into paper for use by the U.S. Navy.

During the excavation of Aztec Ruins, aboriginal hairbrushes made from the pointed ends of yucca leaves were discovered. Strips of banana yucca leaves or whole leaves from the narrowleaf varieties were employed to make paintbrushes and to weave baskets, bags, mats, and tapestry at many Ancestral Puebloan villages. Perhaps the single most universal use was in manufacturing sandals. The 406 sandals recovered during the 1970s excavation of Antelope House at Canyon de Chelly showed surprising diversity in heel and toe shape, heel and toe strap

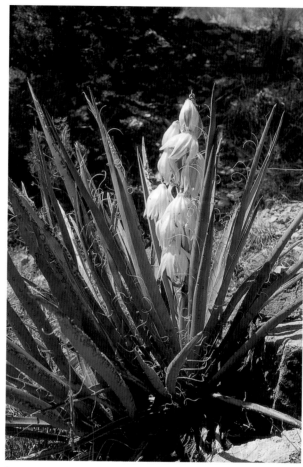

Banana yucca

design, weaving rhythm, weaving technique, and, of course, size. The mix included course-plaited sandals made from banana yucca strips, fine-plaited sandals made from narrowleaf yucca, as well as twined and wicker sandals made from yucca cordage. Some of these woven sandals employed both types of yucca, one in the warp, the other in the woof.

Although the preponderance of evidence for prehistoric use relates to manufacturing, there is plenty to indicate that yucca fruits were an item of the Ancestral Puebloan diet. This is particularly true of the thick, sweet fruit of the banana yucca, which could have been eaten green, although it was more likely dried and stored for use in winter. This tradition has been carried on by direct descendants, the Hopi, who today bake the fruit in earthen ovens. All other native peoples of the Four Corners region, including the Ute Mountain Utes, the Jicarilla Apache, and the Navajo, have collected and eaten these fruits as well as the smaller ones from narrowleaf yucca plants. Yucca fruit pods taste a bit like summer squash, while the flower petals, which are also edible, have a lettuce like flavor.

Loaded with saponin, a well-known lathering substance, the large root of the various yuccas has been the principal source of soap for Indians living throughout the Southwest, both past and present. When pounded, the roots froth with suds. In the old days yucca root suds undoubtedly were employed for all manner of cleaning jobs; hair shampoo stands out as the most enduring use. Among other native peoples, the Navajo say a yucca shampoo will make your hair long, shiny, and black, and several Navajo ceremonies incorporate yucca washings. Many traditional Navajos prefer yucca over commercial soaps to wash wool yarn for their elegant rugs, and yucca suds are used by some Jicarilla Apaches to clean wild plant materials woven into baskets.

Not many medicinal applications are associated with yucca, but the Hopi have used its crushed roots for a strong laxative and to cure baldness; Navajo people use the roots in a medicinal capacity in connection with childbirth.

GREASEWOOD

Goosefoot family
(*Sarcobatus vermiculatus*)

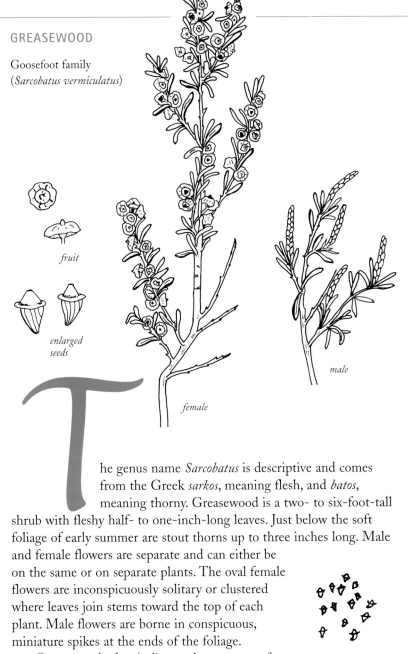

fruit

*enlarged
seeds*

female

male

The genus name *Sarcobatus* is descriptive and comes from the Greek *sarkos*, meaning flesh, and *batos*, meaning thorny. Greasewood is a two- to six-foot-tall shrub with fleshy half- to one-inch-long leaves. Just below the soft foliage of early summer are stout thorns up to three inches long. Male and female flowers are separate and can either be on the same or on separate plants. The oval female flowers are inconspicuously solitary or clustered where leaves join stems toward the top of each plant. Male flowers are borne in conspicuous, miniature spikes at the ends of the foliage.

Greasewood often indicates the presence of saline or alkaline soils. It grows profusely in Chaco Canyon and is

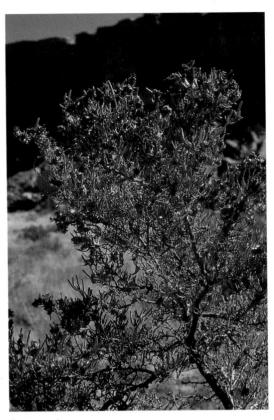
Greasewood

codominant with salt-bush along the drive to Pueblo Bonito. Look for it on the grounds at Aztec Ruins also.

Greasewood remains collected from nearly every prehistoric site in Chaco indicate that it was a construction material, used mainly for lintels, and fuel, especially in the later years of occupation when other woods were less available (Mollie S. Toll, personal communication, 1996). Copious amounts of the pollen have been recovered from these sites. At Antelope House in Canyon de Chelly, greasewood was made into spindle shafts for spinning fibers into yarn, batten rods, and finishing needles.Other items made from greasewood were digging sticks, stirring sticks, scrapers, and awls, along with various ceremonial objects. But the most significant find from Antelope House was thirty-four arrow points and sixty-six shafts that probably were arrow point blanks. *Very* tough wood.

Historic accounts of greasewood verify its hardness. The Hopi consider it the best kind of wood for carving two-foot-long, boomerang-shaped sticks for killing rabbits and for digging or planting sticks similar to those found in prehistoric sites. It is also the favored wood for kiva fires because, when it is dry, it burns with a bright sparkling flame.

Many Navajo tools made of greasewood were similar to those made by the Hopi. In this category are awls, knitting needles, war bows, bird snares, and corn-planting sticks. Some groups of Navajo ate greasewood fruits in the past, and in the vicinity of Chaco, where there is so much of it today, Navajo still collect it for food. They also used it as part of a dye plant formula for creating red, yellow, and blue hues.

Until recently, the Ute Mountain Ute did their own tanning of hides. Those intended for women's garments were left white. Hides used for men's clothing or for utilitarian purposes, such as tepee covers or storage bags, were hung on a tripod over a green greasewood fire for a final smoking. This procedure turned the hides yellow, but by using other types of wood in the fire they were able to vary the color.

Utes also used greasewood for the foreshafts of fish spears, while other tribal groups used it to tip composite arrows made of common reed.

The only medicinal applications of greasewood come from the Navajo, who chew the plant and apply it to the stings of bees, wasps, and ants. It also has been utilized by Navajo in childbirth ceremonies. Fifty years ago a pharmaceutical company found that greasewood contains an effective antioxidant, and for a short time this was being extracted on a large scale in southern New Mexico. Antioxidants are now manufactured synthetically. Although greasewood is certainly plentiful throughout the Southwest, we have heard of no other commercial applications.

FOURWING SALTBUSH

Goosefoot family
(*Atriplex canescens*)

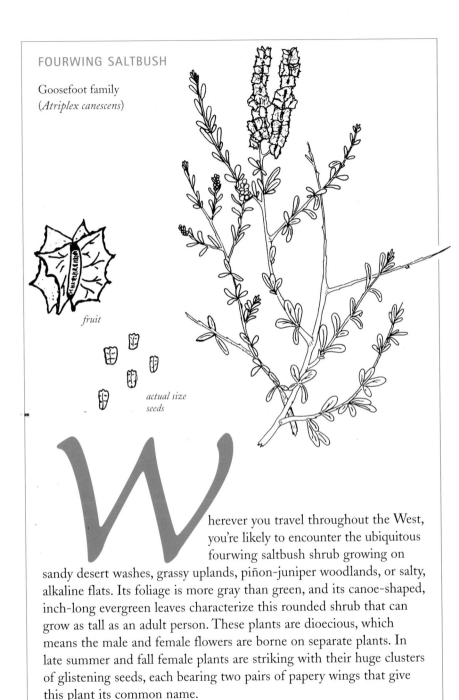

fruit

*actual size
seeds*

Wherever you travel throughout the West, you're likely to encounter the ubiquitous fourwing saltbush shrub growing on sandy desert washes, grassy uplands, piñon-juniper woodlands, or salty, alkaline flats. Its foliage is more gray than green, and its canoe-shaped, inch-long evergreen leaves characterize this rounded shrub that can grow as tall as an adult person. These plants are dioecious, which means the male and female flowers are borne on separate plants. In late summer and fall female plants are striking with their huge clusters of glistening seeds, each bearing two pairs of papery wings that give this plant its common name.

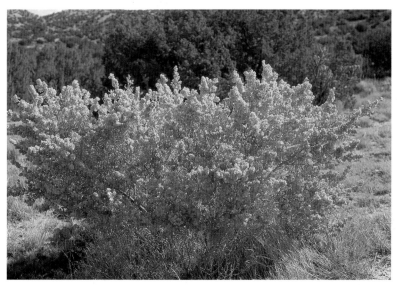
Fourwing saltbush

Fourwing saltbush is especially abundant on the floor of Chaco Canyon, but you'll also find it along the trails at Aztec Ruins, Hovenweep, and Canyon de Chelly. Most of Mesa Verde is too high and forested for the plant, but it does grow there in a few woodland openings.

Saltbush was highly valued during Ancestral Puebloan times. Seeds regularly turn up in desiccated human feces recovered from these sites. At Antelope House in Canyon de Chelly, the prehistoric occupants made brushes with shredded saltbush limbs. It is thought to have been a major source of fuel for Chacoans and even earlier peoples during the Archaic period.

The Hopi continued the tradition of collecting saltbush wood for fuel until the introduction of the metal axe, which facilitated a shift from shrub to tree fuels. Hopi still consider saltbush one of the four shrubs prescribed for their kiva fires. Tradition also calls for their mixing saltbush wood ash with blue cornmeal to provide the alkali necessary for maintaining the color when it is used to make blue piki wafer-bread. The people of Hano, refugees from Rio Grande pueblos who settled on Hopi First Mesa in the 1700s to escape Spanish perse-cution, had a slightly different dye use for saltbush ashes. They stirred them into their dough in order to turn it from purplish gray, the natural color of meal ground from blue kernels, to greenish blue.

Probably all Indians living in the Four Corners once collected saltbush seeds for food. Southern Paiute people were recorded as having ground the seeds of fourwing and two other species of saltbush to make a mush or bread. The Navajo parched and ground the seeds to make flour.

Navajo medicinal uses seem endless. Plant parts were ingested as a home remedy for eating discomfort, while the roots might be boiled in a sweat bath for stomach pain. Leaves and roots are ground to concoct a cough medicine, roots for a toothache, and leaves for snuff, as well as for a poultice for ant bites. Then for hair tonic, leaf and stem ashes are rubbed into the scalp.

The Navajo produce several shades of yellow dye by boiling saltbush leaves and blossoms with raw alum. Wool yarn is then added to this mixture and boiled up to three hours. The Hopi once sprinkled saltbush ashes on buckskin moccasins that had been painted a deep red, which was derived from mountain-mahogany or alder bark dye, in order to bring out the color.

Barberry family
(*Berberis repens*)

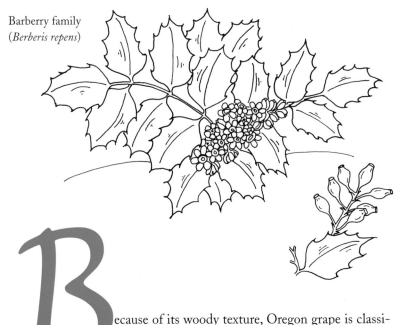

Because of its woody texture, Oregon grape is classified as a shrub, but it's a diminutive, low-growing one, often hugging the ground in shady ponderosa pine or mixed conifer forests. Clusters of bright yellow flowers in spring ripen into blue-black berries in late summer and fall. This plant is best recognized by its compound leaves made up of three to nine paired leaflets, each with prickly, hollylike margins, that turn a deep crimson in fall. When you visit Mesa Verde, you are sure to see Oregon grape along the trail to Spruce Tree House.

Oregon grape is well known as a source of medicine. Both the dark yellow roots and the stem bark contain the chemical berberin, a strong alkaloid that can bestow various beneficial effects. In Navajo country the people produce a tonic from boiled leaves and twigs to alleviate the effects of rheumatism or a lotion to treat scorpion bites, while a tea from the roots is said to be an effective laxative or emetic, depending upon the strength of the brew. Some Navajo living in the Monument Valley region of northern Arizona consider this plant a cure-all for a variety of ailments.

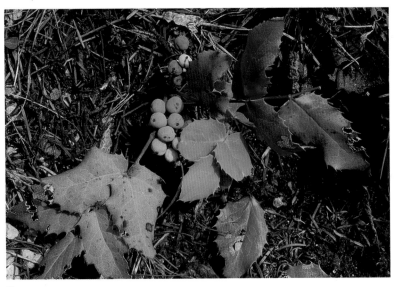
Oregon grape

Various Rio Grande Puebloans drink a tea brewed from plant parts to strengthen their blood, and the Hopi collect its yellow roots for ceremonial use.

Oregon grape berries are tart but not poisonous and no doubt have played at least a minor role in the diet of native people living in the Four Corners region. One early food reference comes from the Southern Paiute Indians who once occupied much territory in southern Utah and northern Arizona. These people ate the berries of the related Fremont barberry (*Berberis fremontii*) shrub and sometimes ground them into a mush. There are to date no archaeological records for Oregon grape in the Four Corners region.

Lydia Pesata, who has been weaving beautiful baskets for more than thirty years and is one of the few living Jicarilla Apache weavers to rely solely on native plants for making her dyes, collects the roots of Oregon grape, then boils them down to produce a pale yellow hue. She also seeks out the roots of a related shrub, Fendler barberry (*B. fendleri*), to achieve a golden color. Navajo weavers make a yellow basket dye from Oregon grape, but their concoction utilizes all of the plant parts excepting the berries.

CLIFF FENDLERBUSH

Saxifrage family
(*Fendlera rupicola*)

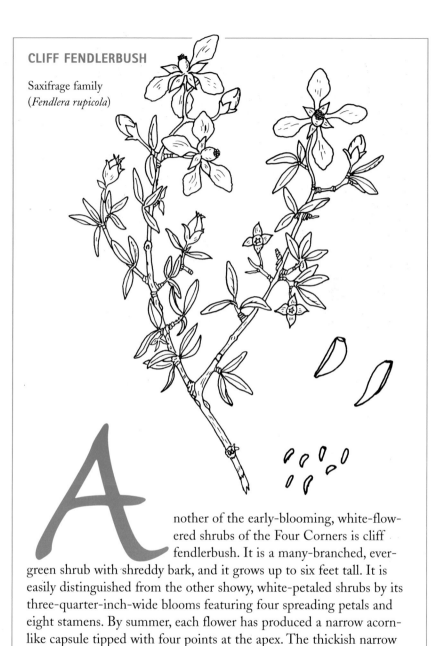

Another of the early-blooming, white-flowered shrubs of the Four Corners is cliff fendlerbush. It is a many-branched, evergreen shrub with shreddy bark, and it grows up to six feet tall. It is easily distinguished from the other showy, white-petaled shrubs by its three-quarter-inch-wide blooms featuring four spreading petals and eight stamens. By summer, each flower has produced a narrow acorn-like capsule tipped with four points at the apex. The thickish narrow leaves have prominent midribs and come in pairs or in clusters.

Cliff fendlerbush grows on rocky slopes in wooded areas; in fact, the scientific name for this species, *rupicola*, translates to "lover of

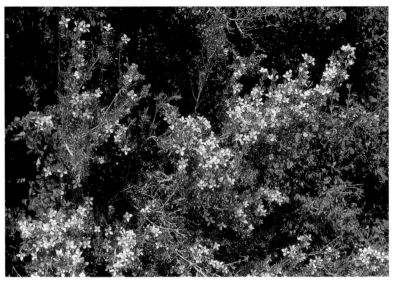
Cliff fendlerbush

rocks." Look for it growing anywhere at Mesa Verde, Hovenweep, or Canyon de Chelly.

Fendlerbush stems tend to be straight, smooth, and nontapered, and its pliable wood hardens when heated by fire. Thus, this was one of the more important woods for the Ancestral Puebloans in manufacturing arrow shafts and points, as well as various tools such as awls and planting sticks. At Canyon de Chelly, where cliff fendlerbush has grown plentifully for at least the past millennium, limb shafts were used to fashion rods for traditional weaving looms and also to make needles for finishing woven products.

The Hopi still collect this shrub for ceremonial purposes; the Navajo use plant parts boiled with juniper berries and piñon buds for purification before some of their ceremonies. Navajo once pounded the inner bark into a pulp and mixed it with water for a medicine to treat certain poisons.

The record shows that Navajos also used cliff fendlerbush for weaving forks, knitting needles, and other articles requiring hard wood. They, too, made arrows from it, and it is probable that other tribes that have inhabited the Four Corners region for centuries did so as well.

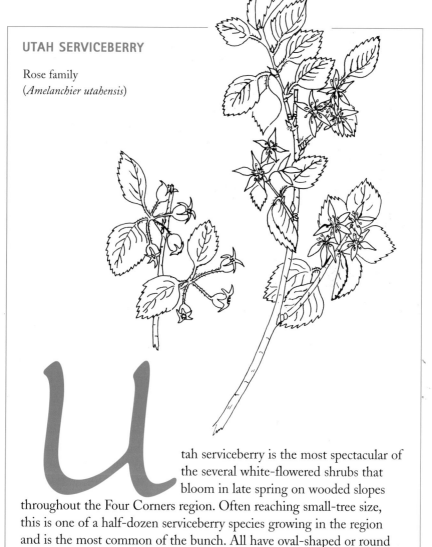

UTAH SERVICEBERRY

Rose family
(*Amelanchier utahensis*)

Utah serviceberry is the most spectacular of the several white-flowered shrubs that bloom in late spring on wooded slopes throughout the Four Corners region. Often reaching small-tree size, this is one of a half-dozen serviceberry species growing in the region and is the most common of the bunch. All have oval-shaped or round leaves with teeth on the margins. The fragrant, five-petaled flowers come in a cluster of three to six blooms at the ends of short branches. By midsummer serviceberry shrubs produce mature bluish-black fruits that are shaped like tiny apples.

The collection of these fruits for food dates to the era of the Ancestral Puebloans. Hopi and Rio Grande Puebloan descendants continue to gather "Indian apples" for the table. The fruits, eaten raw or cooked or dried for winter consumption, were a favorite item

among the Ute and the Southern Paiute.
Early Anglo settlers used the fruit for pies
and puddings and to make pemmican, a
concentrated food item prepared as an emergency ration.

Navajos, too, collect and eat the fruits,
and, not unexpectedly, they have found several medicinal applications for serviceberry,
which is one of their many Life Medicines.
With its emetic action, Navajo people
employ it to treat stomachaches and nausea;
animal bites and skin irritations are treated

enlarged seeds

actual size seeds

with these fruits
as well.

Because service-
berry wood is hard
and heavy, it was ideal
for making a variety
of implements. The
archaeological records
from Mesa Verde and
Canyon de Chelly
show that it was used
to fashion planting
sticks, hoes, arrow
points, and rods
employed in weaving.
Indeed, the shrub is
common at these
sites today.

Serviceberry limbs
were preferred by the
Southern Paiute and
Ute Indians for creat-
ing a number of tools,
including digging

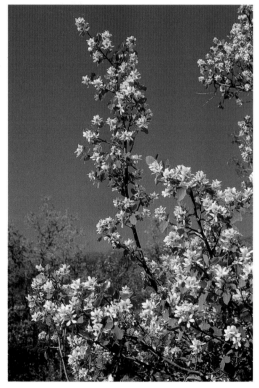
Utah serviceberry

sticks, and arrows. The process Ute craftsmen used to make early bows is described in *Great Basin*, Volume 11 of *Handbook of North American Indians*:"Arrows, both single and composite, 22 to 24 inches long, were made using serviceberry and other hardwoods. Composite arrows were made with cane (i.e. common reed) mainshafts and hardwood foreshafts tipped by sharpening with stone points or with crossed sticks for birds" (Callaway et al. 1986). To remove the bark from a green serviceberry stem, it was first run through a hole in a bone wrench.

The Ute carved single- and double-curved bows from serviceberry wood and made snowshoes with it as well, often in combination with willow or threeleaf sumac. Apache Indians living in east-central Arizona once used the peeled branches to form the uprights for their large carrying baskets.

It is said that there is a dye use for the fruit, but the authors have been unable to track it.

Rose family
(*Rosa woodsii*)

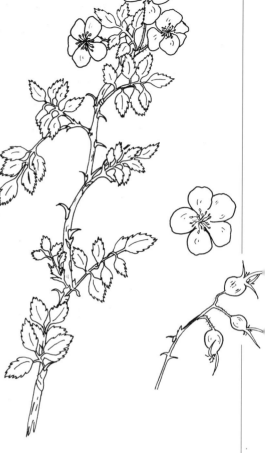

nlike cultivated roses, which have showy blossoms, the first part of a wild rose to catch your attention is likely to be its thorns. Politely called prickles in some plant books, they can be straight or curved, sparse or dense, and quite stout. Wild rose leaves have from five to nine serrated leaflets opposite one another along a common axis, with the odd leaflet at the end; five pink to rose-purple flower petals surround numerous yellow stamens. They bloom from May through June with single, perfect flowers or in clus-

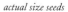

actual size seeds

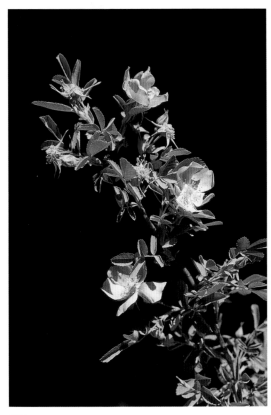
Wild rose

ters on the stem. The red fruit, called a hip, is round or nearly so. Small animals relish rose hips.

Wild roses are common to this continent as well as to Europe. Throughout the southwestern United States, this shrub is found in wet and dry habitats, in valleys and on slopes, on the plains and in the mountains. Wild rose can be readily seen at Mesa Verde along the road to the museum and at Spruce Tree House, at Aztec Ruins, and in ponderosa pine forests across Four Corners country. These useful shrubs are absent from Chaco Canyon.

That rose hips are high in vitamin C is well known; perhaps less well known is that the seeds contain large amounts of the essential E vitamin. When available, rose hips are still sought by all tribes of the Four Corners region. Usually they are collected by women and children and eaten out of hand as a snack. Ute Mountain Ute used to prepare some of their harvest by mashing the hips with or without the seeds, drying them in the sun, and storing them in bags.

Rose hip tea is popular among many people, and the petals were steeped in water and used for fragrance by pioneer women. However, neither the casual drinking of rose tea nor its use as a fragrance is recorded in the ethnobotanical literature covering our area, nor was it mentioned in any of our interviews. Medicinal uses of rose petals have been reported from several Rio Grande Pueblos as treatment for stomach pains, toothaches, sore throats, and wounds. Navajo also have made medicine from it.

The Ute had interesting applications for wild rose other than for food. They made arrows with the stems by first wrenching the stems through holes in bone pieces and, in later times, through holes in cans. This action stripped the stem of its bark and thorns, as did rolling the stem between rocks. This method was used for making arrows out of other thorny shrubs. Utes also made pipe stems from rosewood and smoked the inner bark.

Roses are sometimes implicated in hay fever, but only the old-fashioned, fragrant, domesticated rose. Probably people put their noses right into them. Since they are insect-pollinated and the pollen is not airborne, it is unlikely that wild roses are much of a nuisance. Those we have explored with our noses have little or no fragrance.

MOUNTAIN-MAHOGANY

Rose family
(*Cercocarpus montanus*)

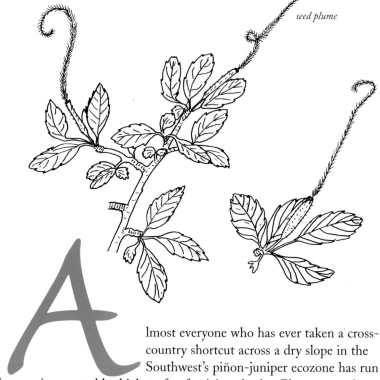

seed plume

Almost everyone who has ever taken a cross-country shortcut across a dry slope in the Southwest's piñon-juniper ecozone has run into an impenetrable thicket of unforgiving shrubs. Chances are the offending obstacle was a stand of mountain-mahogany, a shrub that grows to six feet tall or higher. Inch-long wedge-shaped leaves are toothed on the upper margins only. The petal-less flowers are inconspicuous, but up to three-inch long, delicate, silky plumes remain attached to the fruit capsule and give mountain-mahogany a distinctive silvery look from late summer on into winter.

This shrub is common along the ruins loop roads at Mesa Verde and the rim roads at Canyon de Chelly. At Chaco it grows near Pueblo Alto.

Mountain-mahogany is dense and tough; indeed, the word for mountain-mahogany in Navajo means "wood heavy as stone." Long

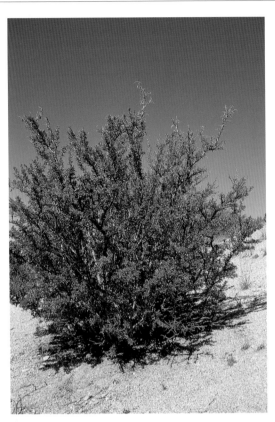
Mountain-mahogany

before Navajo people arrived in the Four Corners region, the wood was used by the Ancestral Puebloans and their predecessors in diverse ways. An ancient hoe made from this wood was among the woody artifacts recovered from Wetherill Mesa at Mesa Verde National Park, while at Antelope House in Canyon de Chelly National Monument mountain-mahogany was employed by at least one ancient weaver to fashion a batten for tightening woven material. It was commonly used as a roofing material.

Mountain-mahogany has been one of three woods utilized by the Ute Indians to craft sinew-backed, double-curved hunting bows. The bow wood was first made flexible by soaking it in water; then it was staked on the ground to give the bow its permanent shape. Navajos, Hopis, and Rio Grande Puebloans traditionally selected this wood to make a variety of implements, including digging sticks, tool handles, and weaving gear, and it is a favorite material for crafting Navajo dice.

The red bark of mountain-mahogany roots is boiled in water to produce a reddish-brown pigment used by both Navajos and Hopis to dye wool. Various shades of brown ranging from orange- and rose-brown to a creamy tan can be produced by adding to the mountain-mahogany mixture other wild plant products, such as juniper ashes, prickly pear fruits, Indian tea stems, alder bark, or lichens. For dying strips of sumac or willow to weave into her baskets, the root is boiled by Jicarilla Apache artisan Lydia Pesata. She informed us that she collects the roots in fall when the reddish-brown color is strongest, and that the runners closest to the central root system make the best concoction.

Navajo Indians have especially strong ties to this shrub. Besides the implement and dye uses cited above, mountain-mahogany roots are considered to be one of the Life Medicines. The bark is also used medicinally by at least one other group of people. The Paiute Indians of southern Utah have been known to brew a tea from the leaves of this plant. The beverage probably had a medicinal connection, because the tea really doesn't compare in taste with those made from several other wild plants.

CLIFFROSE

Rose family
(*Cowania stansburiana*)

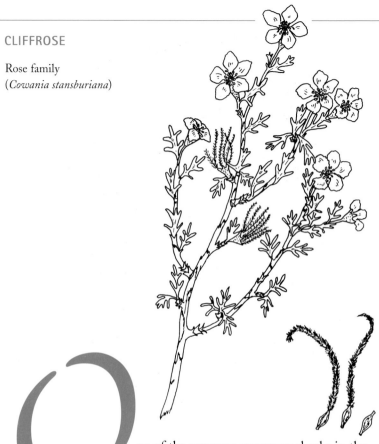

One of the common evergreen shrubs in the Four Corners piñon-juniper ecozone, cliffrose grows to six feet tall and has small, mostly five-lobed, wedge-shaped leaves that turn under at the margins. The cream-colored, sweet-smelling flowers of early summer produce long, showy, white- to rose-colored plumes in the fall. Cliffrose is easily confused with bitterbrush (*Purshia tridentata*), which grows in similar settings, and the two plants can hybridize. Bitterbrush has yellower flowers, and its leaves are always three-lobed. Plant uses for the two species seem to be identical, and most contemporary Indians do not distinguish between them.

Cliffrose is ubiquitous at Canyon de Chelly and Hovenweep and can be found along the trail to Pueblo Alto at Chaco. Bitterbrush, also

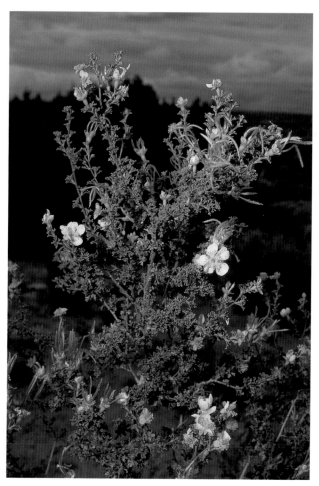

Cliffrose

known as antelope brush, grows abundantly at Mesa Verde and the adjacent Ute Mountain Tribal Park.

Cliffrose, along with bitterbrush, has a long history as a useful plant because of its stout and often straight branches, its shreddy bark, and its leaves' chemical content from which it acquired its common name, qui-nine-bush. Both Hopi and Navajo ingest the bitter leaves to induce vomiting in the event of stomachache or nausea, and both use a leaf broth to wash wounds and treat skin problems. The leaves also may be used for a cough syrup, and Ute Indians use a potion made from inner bark as an eyewash.

This is a major Navajo dye plant. A gold dye for wool is obtained by boiling the twigs and leaves for two hours, adding raw alum (obtained from natural exposures at the base of cliffs in several places on the reservation) for a mordant, then boiling the wool in this mixture for another two hours. When mixed with powdered juniper branches, pounded cliffrose leaves and stems make a tan dye.

The cliffrose's straight limbs were one of several plants whose parts were used by both Hopi and Navajo Indians to fashion arrow shafts. Both tribes stripped the bark and shredded it for cradleboard padding or pillow stuffing. Harry Walters, chairperson for the Center of Diné Studies at the Navajo Community College in Tsaili, Arizona, told us that cliffrose bark is *the* material for baby matting because it doesn't give a child a rash like Utah juniper matting does and it effectively absorbs urine. Interestingly, the Navajo word for baby cradle and cliffrose is the same.

With so many historic uses for cliffrose in the Four Corners region, you might expect it to be among the plants used by the Ancestral Puebloans, but for some reason it isn't. This may be because charcoal from plants in the rose family is difficult to distinguish at the species level. We were able to track down only one reference to a small amount of cliffrose/bitterbrush charcoal recovered from a single site at Chaco, where its prehistoric use was undeterminable.

THREELEAF SUMAC

Sumac family
(*Rhus trilobata*)

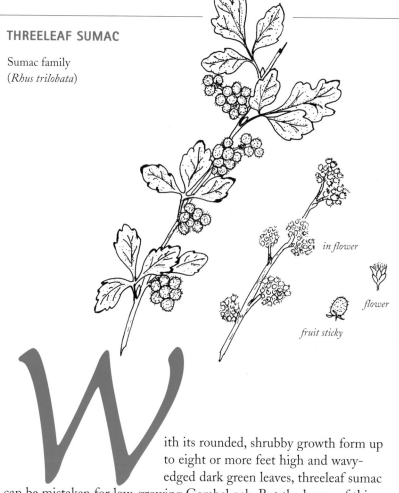

in flower

flower

fruit sticky

With its rounded, shrubby growth form up to eight or more feet high and wavy-edged dark green leaves, threeleaf sumac can be mistaken for low-growing Gambel oak. But the leaves of this plant are not merely lobed, they are strongly three-parted, and the tiny pale yellow flowers that appear in early spring produce sticky, hairy, pea-sized reddish berries rather than acorns. Like some of the eastern deciduous oaks, threeleaf sumac turns a deep red in the fall.

Thickets or single shrubs of threeleaf sumac are widespread on open slopes throughout the piñon-juniper ecozone. Look for it at Aztec Ruins and Hovenweep, along the Chapin Mesa loop roads at Mesa Verde, and on the trail to Pueblo Alto at Chaco.

The track record for human use of this shrub in our area goes back at least two thousand years. Remains of the berries are found in coprolites from Ancestral Puebloan sites throughout the Four Corners region. Perhaps the most numerous documented findings for prehistoric uses come from the excavation of Antelope House in Canyon de Chelly in the 1970s. There plant parts were being eaten around A.D. 1200, and sumac wood or its fibers was being crafted into baskets, snowshoes, loom rods and anchors, arrow points and shafts, digging sticks, scrapers, awls, and a multitude of ceremonial objects. A number

enlarged seed

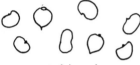

actual size seeds

of damaged ceramic pots that had been repaired by winding strips of sumac through repair holes drilled at the point of the crack were unearthed here. Exploiting the tough and limber qualities of sumac twigs for pot repair probably was an extension of its many applications by basket-making people.

Clearly, the basket-making tradition for threeleaf sumac was continued by descendants of the Ancestral Puebloans, as evidenced by Hopi baskets made from this material right up to the present day.

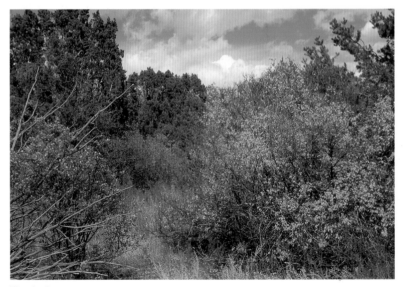

Threeleaf sumac

Along with willow, it is the material preferred by virtually all native basket makers who have inhabited the Four Corners, including Navajo, Paiute, Pueblo, Jicarilla Apache, and, of course, the Ute artisans whose baskets are world famous.

Charles Marsh describes the traditional Ute basket-making process in his book, *People of the Shining Mountains*: "The familiar coiled baskets were usually made of squaw brush when the finest quality was desired, while thin willow branches were used for more coarse basketry. Squaw brush was best gathered in the spring when it was soft and supple and was stored until needed. Before weaving, the material was soaked in water to make it more pliable. Sometimes colored designs were woven into the baskets by inserting vegetable-dyed colored strands, and these fine patterns have made the few remaining examples of old Ute basketry very valuable" (Marsh 1982). Squawbush, or squawbrush, is another of the several names for this shrub, and it comes from the fact that Indian women of many tribes preferred it for their basketry.

The high tannin content of sumac branches and leaves has led Hopi weavers to use it in making their natural dye mordants, which are the chemicals used to set the color of a dye and make it insoluble in water. Hopi, Navajo, and Pueblo Indians all mix crushed sumac branchlets and leaves with yellow ocher mineral and piñon pine pitch to produce black pigment for dying wool or baskets. Navajo also use fermented sumac berries to produce an orange-brown dye.

Lemonade-bush is yet another name for this plant, owing to its tart berries that to this day are ground up and mixed with water or tea to create a favorite beverage for almost all native peoples living in the Four Corners area.

Hopi people suffering from tuberculosis once used a combination of sumac roots and piñon pine parts to combat the effects of this disease, while Navajo use pulverized leaves to treat stomachaches and a variety of skin problems. A concoction of sumac berries also has been used by the Navajo as a treatment for hair loss.

WHIPPLE CHOLLA

Cactus family
(*Opuntia whipplei*)

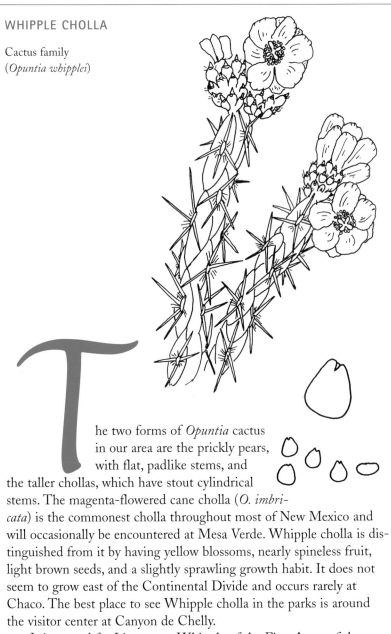

The two forms of *Opuntia* cactus in our area are the prickly pears, with flat, padlike stems, and the taller chollas, which have stout cylindrical stems. The magenta-flowered cane cholla (*O. imbricata*) is the commonest cholla throughout most of New Mexico and will occasionally be encountered at Mesa Verde. Whipple cholla is distinguished from it by having yellow blossoms, nearly spineless fruit, light brown seeds, and a slightly sprawling growth habit. It does not seem to grow east of the Continental Divide and occurs rarely at Chaco. The best place to see Whipple cholla in the parks is around the visitor center at Canyon de Chelly.

It is named for Lieutenant Whipple of the First Army of the West, who collected it near Zuni in 1846. Common to valleys and

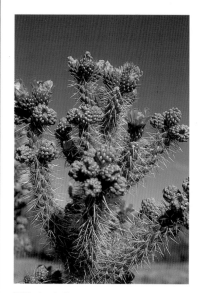
Whipple cholla

plains from 4,500 to 7,000 feet elevation in southern Utah and northern Arizona, Whipple cholla blooms from June to October.

While cane cholla has edible fruits and seeds and is sufficiently closely related to Whipple cholla to hybridize, it is not at all clear if the common Four Corners cholla, *O. whipplei*, has edible parts.

While cholla seeds are known to have been an important part of the diet in Ancestral Puebloan times, only in the past few years have ethnobotanists been able to tell the species of excavated seeds apart. It appears that Whipple cholla was either used infrequently

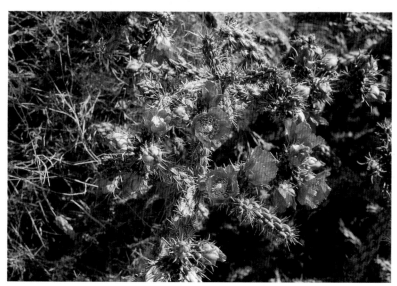
Cane cholla

or not at all prehistorically or was not there to be used. Although cholla pollen and charred buds were recovered at Salmon Ruin near present-day Farmington, and *O. whipplei* is the species growing there now, at the time the site was excavated the seeds of prehistoric *Opuntia* could not be readily differentiated. A later excavation at nearby Chaco contained only prickly pear, not cholla, cactus seeds.

While it has been reported that the Southern Paiute collected both buds and fruits of Whipple cholla for food, other tribes in the Four Corners tell a different story. Navajo do not eat any part of this cholla, contending it is not edible and perhaps poisonous, yet the Hopi are said to have boiled the fruit with squash as a food. Their close relatives, the Zuni Puebloans, also were recorded as having eaten Whipple cholla fruit that was raw or stewed or dried and ground into flour, which was mixed with parched cornmeal and made into mush.

The single medicinal reference comes from the Hopi, who once drank a boiled liquid from a pounded mixture of Whipple cholla and globe-mallow for diarrhea.

BEARBERRY

Heath family
(*Arctostaphylos uva-ursi*)

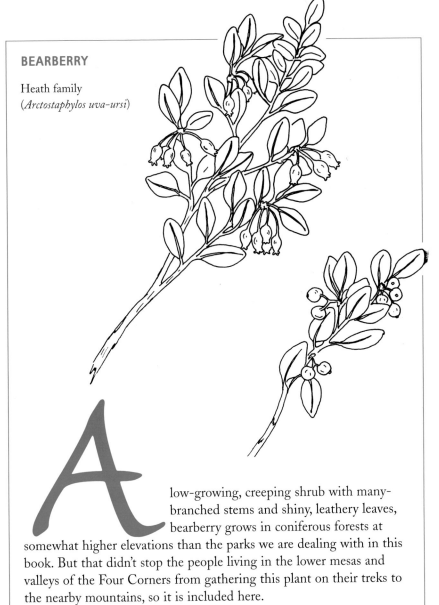

A low-growing, creeping shrub with many-branched stems and shiny, leathery leaves, bearberry grows in coniferous forests at somewhat higher elevations than the parks we are dealing with in this book. But that didn't stop the people living in the lower mesas and valleys of the Four Corners from gathering this plant on their treks to the nearby mountains, so it is included here.

Pink to white, urn-shaped flowers of summer mature into rather tasteless bright red berries in fall. We are not sure of the precise connection of bearberry with bears, but surely there is one, for the scientific name of the genus *Arctostaphylos* comes from the Greek and translates to "bear and grape," while the specific name, *uva-ursi*, is Latin for "grape-bear."

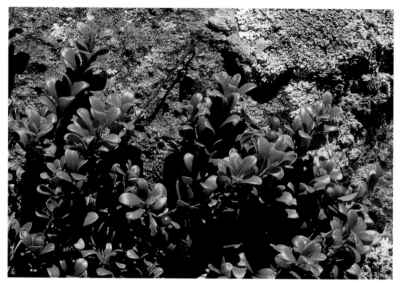
Bearberry

In our region the best-known use for bearberry among various native peoples has been for smoking. All along the Rio Grande, Puebloans have dried the leaves and smoked them plain or, in recent times, mixed the dried leaves with store-bought tobacco. Others, including the Ute and Navajo, formerly used tobacco (*Nicotiana* spp.) collected in the wild as part of the mixture.

Although there are no records indicating that bearberry fruits played any role in the peoples' diet, the fruits of two closely related, tall-growing shrubs found at lower elevations in the Four Corners region definitely were dietary items. Both pointleaf manzanita (*Arctostaphylos pungens*) and green-leaf manzanita (*A. patula*) berries have been consumed, either fresh or dried, by Navajos living in the Canyon de Chelly area in Arizona and by Southern Paiutes from Utah.

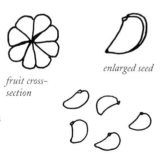
fruit cross-section

enlarged seed

actual size seeds

The leaves of greenleaf manzanita are taken by the Navajo as an emetic to treat stomach problems and also are used for insect bites. We haven't come across local Native American medicinal uses for bearberry, but worldwide, cures using this plant, which is native to Europe and Asia as well as North America, are legion.

The first known use of bearberry was by Welsh physicians in the thirteenth century. Because bearberry leaves have antiseptic, diuretic, and anti-inflammatory qualities, they were once used by American settlers to treat urinary disorders and now are widely taken in Europe and elsewhere for bladder, kidney, and urinary tract problems. At last count, our local health food store offered five different herbal medicine or food supplement products featuring *Arctostaphylos uva-ursi* as the main ingredient.

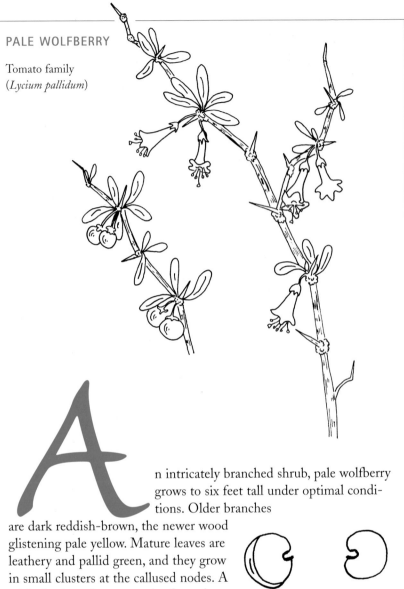

PALE WOLFBERRY

Tomato family
(*Lycium pallidum*)

An intricately branched shrub, pale wolfberry grows to six feet tall under optimal conditions. Older branches are dark reddish-brown, the newer wood glistening pale yellow. Mature leaves are leathery and pallid green, and they grow in small clusters at the callused nodes. A wicked spine often protrudes from these nodes where the branch changes angle. Flowers are inch-long, creamy-green funnels that blossom from May to June. Orange-red berries, ripening in July, resemble miniature tomatoes.

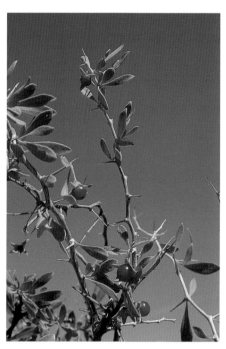
Pale wolfberry

The genus *Lycium* has a curious distribution; it grows from South America to the Southwest in a funnel-shaped pattern, with the Southwest and northern Mexico at the top of the funnel where most species occur. Pale wolfberry is present near the major ruins at all the parks featured in this book and on or nearby many other ruins in the Four Corners region.

The link between pale wolfberry and prehistoric ruins has been known for a long time. It is suspected to have been caused by intentional or inadvertent prehistoric Indian introduction of seeds and subsequent sprouting of plants on nearby disturbed soil. After a pueblo has been abandoned, a constant, hidden reservoir of moisture that collects over decomposing subsurface floors, plazas, or water catchment devices provides ideal habitat for generations of wolfberry shrubs. All of this seems to add up to wolfberry growing where people have carried it and created a suitable habitat. Wolfberry seeds are commonly found in prehistoric sites. At Salmon Ruin seeds were found in some middens and are considered cultural artifacts.

Wolfberry is part of a large and diverse plant family that includes sacred datura, common potato, tobacco, tomatillo, belladonna, petunia, and eggplant. Members of this family have a reputation for at least some part of the various species containing poisonous alkaloids, and it's likely that wolfberry does, too. These chemicals can cause numbing of the flesh, and members of one Rio Grande Pueblo have applied fresh or water-soaked dried wolfberry leaves to cuts. Navajo have used the heated ground-up root for toothaches. At Zuni pieces of the root were soaked in water overnight and then buried near their corn plants to keep the worms from eating the roots. Such applications suggest that wolfberry might have analgesic, antiseptic, and insecticidal properties.

As did other southwestern tribes, Hopi and Navajo ate the ripened sweet berries straight from the shrub or cooked with white clay. "Food clay," a Navajo term, or "potato clay," a Hopi term, was used to take away the bitterness of the potentially poisonous alkaloids or to act as a detoxifier. Native people also dried the fruits for winter when they sometimes boiled them in soup. Hopi on occasion mixed them with cream of potato clay and then ate them with piki bread. Clay is very absorbent and tends to swell with water, filling an empty stomach; indeed, wolfberry was a famine food during the 1863 drought when many Hopi had to leave their homes and live for a time with the Rio Grande Puebloans. Wolfberry is still used in ceremonies. Native peoples do not forget the debt owed some of these ancient food plants.

SNOWBERRY

Honeysuckle family
(*Symphoricarpos* spp.)

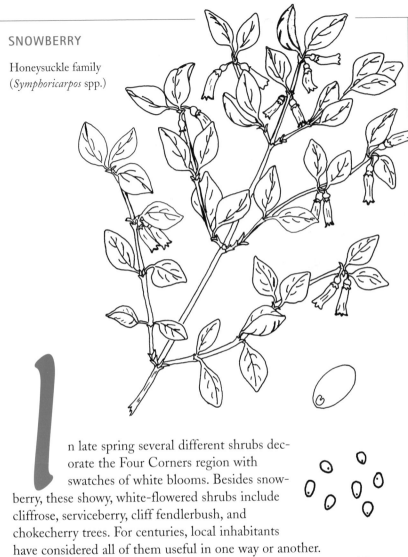

In late spring several different shrubs decorate the Four Corners region with swatches of white blooms. Besides snowberry, these showy, white-flowered shrubs include cliffrose, serviceberry, cliff fendlerbush, and chokecherry trees. For centuries, local inhabitants have considered all of them useful in one way or another.

A number of species of snowberry grow in the Southwest. All are many-branched, medium-sized deciduous shrubs with oval-shaped leaves that have smooth, sometimes slightly lobed edges. The small white-to-pink tubular flowers tipped with four or five lobes are borne in pairs or small clusters and produce white berries toward the end of summer. Most species of snowberry prefer cooler, wetter upland conditions and so are not found in most of the parks covered here, the

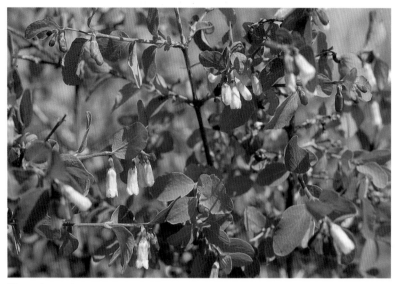

Mountain snowberry

exception being Mesa Verde, where the local species, mountain snowberry (*Symphoricarpos oreophilus*), is plentiful throughout the Morefield Campground but less common in other parts of the park.

Snowberry is considered by most to be a somewhat minor medicine plant. From the literature, it's not always clear which parts of the plant have been used for various treatments. Navajo have used plant parts in some way for sore throats and colds, and snowberry leaves are one of the many plants employed as a pre-ceremony emetic. These shrubs produce acrid-flavored berries that also have been used in historic times as a purge or emetic.

Snowberry roots are associated with treating stomach problems. The leaves once were smoked by Southern Paiute Indians, who also used rods made from snowberry to encircle a baby's cradle.

BROOM SNAKEWEED

Sunflower family
(*Gutierrezia sarothrae*)

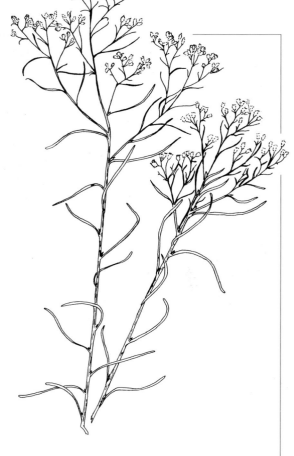

flower
head

In fall the golden globes of broom snakeweed brighten the arid grassy landscape at lower elevations throughout
the Four Corners and beyond. During the rest
of the year this many-stemmed semishrub
growing to a foot or so tall is much less conspicuous. A waxy finish on the dark green foliage is
due to resins contained in the glossy, gland-dotted
leaves. Considered a perennial, individual snakeweed plants normally die after three years or so.

Broom snakeweed grows profusely in most of the
park settings covered in this book. Its leaves contain the
sudsing agent saponin and are toxic to most livestock. Thus,

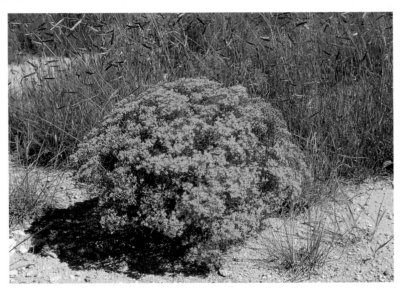

Broom snakeweed

the plant becomes a range pest where selective grazing allows it to increase at the expense of palatable grasses.

Usually snakeweed is not found growing in the immediate vicinity of archaeological ruins. That may be due to its preference for sandy soils, whereas the increase in soil clay resulting from decomposing pueblo walls around old ruins may constitute a barrier to snakeweed survival.

Pueblo Indians have long recognized the medicinal values of this resinous shrub, although specific remedies vary widely from pueblo to pueblo. Medicinal applications include general purification, as well as cures for colds, fever, sores, stomach ailments, eye problems, rheumatism, and rattlesnake bites, as described in the companion volume to this book, *Wild Plants of the Pueblo Province*.

Broom snakeweed figures strongly in the various herbal remedies associated with Hispanic tradition; indeed, the genus is named for Pedro Gutierrez, a nineteenth-century botanist from Madrid. Some of the medicinal uses of snakeweed by Hispanic people in the Southwest undoubtedly originated from their early contacts with Pueblo and other Indians.

Hopi people use snakeweed foliage in a brew to counteract gastrointestinal disturbances, and plant parts occasionally are added to sweet corn prepared for the table, but this second use also may have a medicinal connection. It seems possible that these Hopi applications originated from the small band of northern Rio Grande Tewa-speaking Puebloans who migrated to First Mesa in A.D. 1700 and who have lived in Hopi country ever since.

Broom snakeweed is one of many species of plants considered to be a Life Medicine by Navajo people. Life Medicine herbs are gathered, dried, and saved for future medicinal use around the home or taken on trips for emergencies rather than being picked for immediate purposes. The Navajo utilize snakeweed root to combat stomach problems and leafy parts to treat headaches and nervousness, to heal cuts, or to reduce swelling from insect bites. In Navajoland snakeweed medicine is often administered during childbirth.

Some Navajos are said to use the flowers in concocting a yellow dye, but that use does not seem to be recognized by other Native American craftspeople.

Interestingly, neither snakeweed seeds nor plant parts turn up in prehistoric archaeological settings, probably because the seeds and other parts are virtually indistinguishable from those of many other plants of the sunflower family and so have not been isolated by archaeobotanists. Another reason for its scarcity in prehistoric caches may be that the plant, although indigenous, was not nearly as common as it is today, having increased over the years due to the overgrazing of palatable species and the avoidance of snakeweed by sheep and cattle.

RABBITBRUSH

Sunflower family
(*Chrysothamnus nauseosus*)

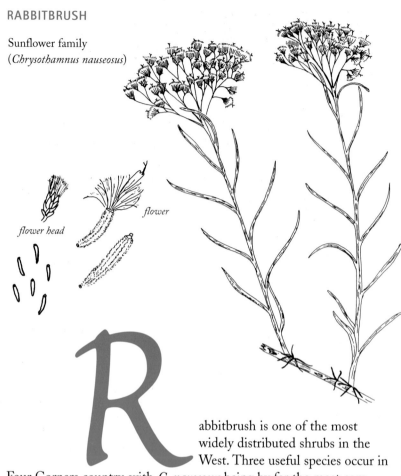

flower head

flower

abbitbrush is one of the most widely distributed shrubs in the West. Three useful species occur in Four Corners country, with *C. nauseosus* being by far the most common. Its gray-green foliage and numerous upright branches reaching four feet tall or more usually give it away; in the fall everyone recognizes rabbitbrush from the rich, gold masses of flowers that cover the rounded shape of each plant.

These shrubs have an affinity for Four Corners roadsides. That's because rabbitbrush needs more moisture than many other shrubs common to the region, a requirement that is satisfied by extra highway surface runoff from summer storms, which effectively doubles annual precipitation absorbed by the soil near the road. Rabbitbrush, known as *chamisa* throughout much of the Southwest, grows in abundance at

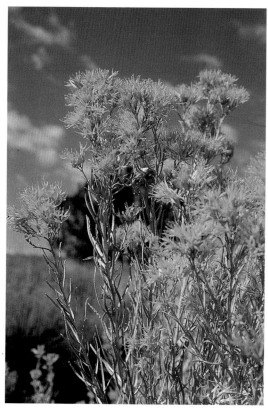
Rabbitbrush

all the parks covered in this book.

One phenomenon likely to strike you is the grape-sized white galls that adorn the stems of so many of these plants. The galls are caused by fruit flies that have laid their eggs on rabbitbrush stems, just as they do on various orchard fruits. A chemical injected into the plant by the fly triggers the plant to grow tumorlike tissue that eventually encases the insect larva. Some botanists claim they can identify the many subspecies of *C. nauseosus* just from the color, shape, and size of their galls, and some suspect that more than one species of fruit fly may be involved.

Proven Ancestral Puebloan use of rabbitbrush is limited to their burning the branches for fuel, although it seems likely that prehistoric people found other ways to benefit from such a common shrub. Plant parts are certainly edible, as attested to by contemporary Navajo, who may add the greens to a stew or concoct a mush or bread from the seeds.

Navajo, of course, found many medicinal uses for these shrubs, including a leaf extract used in cleansing ceremonies and for headaches and root concentrates for colds and internal injuries. The tips of

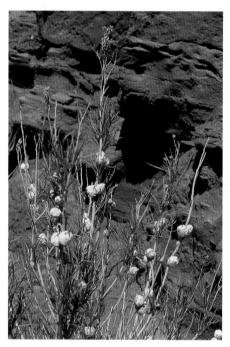
Insect galls on rabbitbrush

these plants have been chewed by the Hopi and applied to boils in order to dry them out.

Hopi also made arrows and wicker mats from the peeled, straight stems, but it is the manufacture of dyes that really distinguishes these plants. Both Hopi and Navajo used rabbitbrush extracts to produce basket, wool, and cotton dyes—the flowers for yellow and bark from the stem for yellow to green. *Hopi Dyes* is an informative book that offers sixteen different recipes for creating different shades of yellow and green dye from rabbitbrush alone or mixed with various mineral pigments or mordants (Colton 1965).

Years ago Francis Elmore described one process used by the Navajo: "To produce a lemon-yellow dye, the flowering tops of the rabbitbrush are boiled for about six hours. Native alum is then heated over a fire until it is reduced to a pasty consistency. These two are then mixed together and the wool put in and allowed to boil for about an hour, or until the desired shade is obtained" (Elmore 1944).

We were unable to locate a traditional Ute Mountain Ute basketmaker to discuss uses of this plant, but Lydia Pesata told us that she uses rabbitbrush stems to make a pale yellow dye for her lovely Jicarilla Apache baskets.

BIG SAGEBRUSH

Sunflower family
(*Artemisia tridentata*)

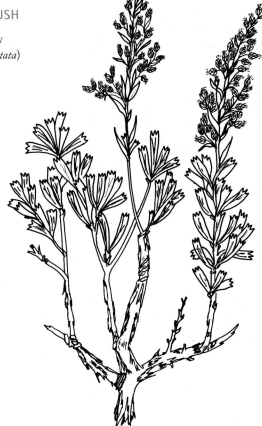

I f not the most common, big sagebrush is certainly more conspicuous than the several other species of sagebrush growing in the Four Corners region. Vast stands of pale gray-turquoise announce the presence of this shrub. Because big sagebrush usually grows in deep, non-saline soils suitable for farming, today in many places these stands are being sectioned into agricultural land.

Even from a distance big sagebrush can be recognized by its smoky color and uniform spacing of plants. Up close its strong turpentine fragrance, especially after a rainstorm, is a dead giveaway. It usually grows from two to five or more feet tall as a dry-looking shrub

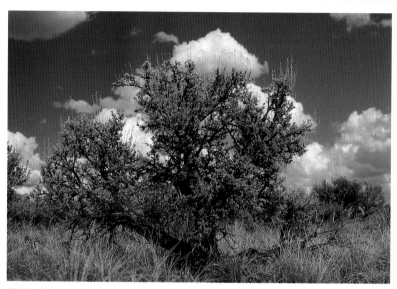

Big sagebrush

with long, soft bark that hangs in shreds. The leaves are about an inch long and wedge-shaped, with three teeth at the end. Flowers are tiny and nondescript. Big sagebrush is abundant in all of the parks covered here except for on the saline-soil floor of Chaco Canyon where grease-wood prevails.

Before the present Ute, Navajo, Apache, and Hopi tribes occupied these lands, the Fremont people who lived north of the Four Corners had developed an industry where much of everything that was woven or crafted from plant material was of big sagebrush. Ancestral Puebloans also used the bark and other parts of the plant. On the Colorado Plateau and southward, sagebrush was one of the principal shrub fuels during Archaic, Ancestral Puebloan, and early historic times.

Sagebrush flowers, seeds, and leaves have been detected in copro-lites from many Ancestral Puebloan sites, including those at Mesa Verde, and in enough quantity to suggest all were minor components of prehistoric diets and not just taken occasionally for medicinal pur-poses. Indeed, sagebrush leaves are a good source of iron and vitamin C and in later years were eaten by the Southern Paiute during times of shortage. However, a body of evidence indicates that sagebrush has poisonous properties that can cause birth defects in animals but can be effective as an antihelminthic. The ancients probably knew how much could be ingested for food with no aftereffects and to what degree it could be used to kill intestinal worms without killing the patient.

In more recent times plant parts have been collected principally for medicinal and ceremonial purposes. The leaves are used to combat digestive problems, headaches, and colds and as a general stimulant by the Hopi, who regard big sagebrush as being more potent than related species of *Artemisia* that grow on their reservation.

The Navajo use a boiled extract of leaves for coughs, colds, headaches, stomachaches, and fevers, as well as for pain during child delivery. It is one of the Navajo Life Medicines and is highly revered by these people. Navajo weavers boil the leaves and twigs to produce various shades of yellow and gold dye.

Ethnographer Anne Smith recorded the Utes' many uses of these plants. She wrote of sacks of woven sagebrush bark lined with dry grass filled with food and placed in storage caches. Wicks, or "slow matches," made of twisted or braided sagebrush bark (and occasionally juniper bark), one to three inches in diameter and about a yard long, were carried when traveling. "Women wore skirts of twined sagebrush bark, and both men and women in winter wore a poncho type of shirt of the same material.... Leggings were also made of twined sagebrush bark or the legs were wrapped with sagebrush bark to protect them from the cold. Sagebrush bark was used for sandals in lieu of anything better... or placed inside sandals made from muskrat or beaver hides" (Smith 1974).

GRASSES

INDIAN RICEGRASS

Grass family
(*Oryzopsis hymenoides*)

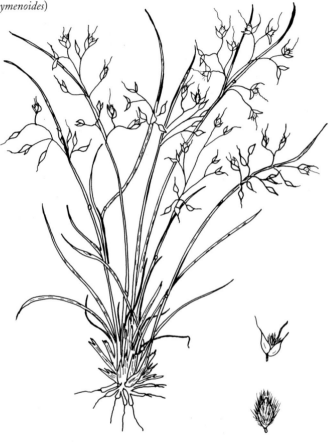

In any season this is one of the easiest grasses to identify in the field. Each plant consists of a dense clump of narrow, tightly rolled leaves with stems up to two feet tall that give the plant a lacy appearance. By late May or June, mature plants produce clusters of solitary large seeds, each encased in a pair of bracts resembling a tiny bell, a dead giveaway. After dropping their seeds, the bell-shaped bracts remain through the following spring.

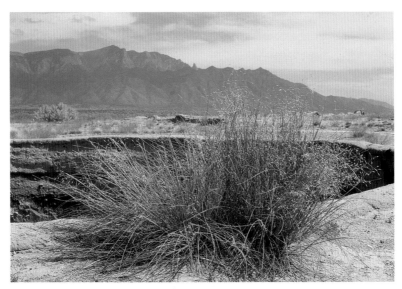
Indian ricegrass

Indian ricegrass, also known as Indian millet, thrives on sandy soils in open places throughout the Southwest except in the higher mountains and driest deserts. It is abundant in all the parks covered here.

The seeds of this plant have comprised a food staple for native peoples living in the Four Corners region at least since Archaic times. The distinctive seeds and seedcases have been identified in coprolites throughout the Ancestral Puebloan realm, surfacing at most of the major sites where ethnobotanical techniques have been employed, including those at Salmon Ruin, Chimney Rock Mesa, and Canyon de Chelly.

At Mesa Verde, where the plants thrive today on decomposed sandstone soils on mesa tops, several clumps of Indian ricegrass with singed ends were recovered during the excavation of Long House and Mug House. But on the floor of Chaco Canyon, where the soil tends to be more of a claylike silt rather than sand, Indian ricegrass is not quite as common. That may have been the case, too, during Chaco's heyday a thousand years ago, for ricegrass seed occurs somewhat less frequently than that of dropseed grass (*Sporobolus* spp.) in the mix of prehistoric plant remains that have been examined there.

Ricegrass seeds are not particularly high in starch or sugar compared with wheat or other cultivated grains. However, an ounce of seed does yield about 120 calories.

Various Indian tribes included ricegrass seeds in their diet right into the past century. Hopis and Navajos used to harvest and process the seeds for the table, as did the Southern Paiute Indians living in the Four Corners region.

One of the best descriptions of the entire procedure comes from Jan Pettit, who interviewed Ute tribal elders:

> Seeds were gathered by brushing the seeds into baskets or onto pieces of buckskin with willow branches or small woven fans. A large conical basket was carried on the back where the seeds were placed from time to time. It would take two to three hours to fill a basket.
>
> Seeds were parched on flat basketry trays by placing a handful or two of powdered charcoal or ash over them. The ashes and seed were then tossed in the air so that the chaff would be carried away by the wind or blown away by mouth. A day's labor could result in about a fourth of a bushel of clean seeds.
>
> The seeds were usually roasted in a tray in which hot coals and the seeds were tossed back and forth for ten or fifteen minutes. This process pops the shells leaving a clean white grain. A nourishing hot grain cereal could be made by cooking the seeds in boiling water in a basket pot (Pettit 1990).

COMMON REED

Grass family
(*Phragmites communis*)

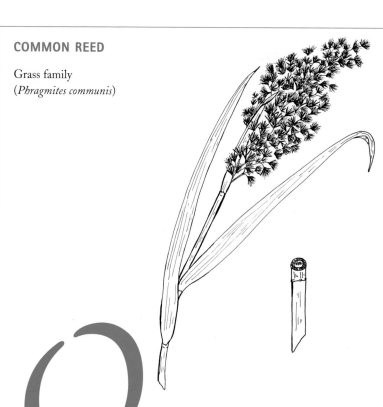

One of three *Phragmites* species in the world, common reed is the most cosmopolitan of the freshwater reeds. Present on nearly every continent, it is a stout, perennial grass that grows from thick, creeping rootstocks called *rhizomes*. The hollow stems can reach ten feet tall, and a flower plume at the top of the plant adds another fifteen to twenty inches. Leaves are broad, flat, and long. Common reed grows along streams and ditches, in ponds, and in many of the same places as cattails. In fact, some ethnobotanists wonder if the common reed might be part of a wetland complex of plants whose distribution partly depended upon the habits of ancient people. This reed thrives along the valley floor in Canyon de Chelly and is occasionally seen near seeps and springs at Mesa Verde and Hovenweep. At Ute Mountain Tribal Park you'll find it growing along the Mancos River, but it no longer occurs in Chaco Wash, although it surely did a thousand years ago when the canyon was occupied.

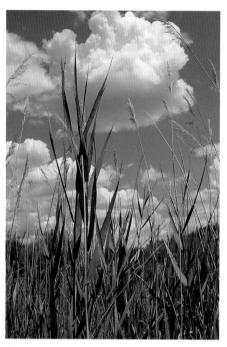
Common reed

Roots, shoots, and seeds of common reed have been used throughout the world for cooked food. In the Southwest and Mexico, reeds are known as *carrizo*, and cordage, nets, mats, screens, and thatching are still occasionally made from them. Artifacts made from common reed have been discovered at nearly all the major ruins in the Four Corners region. It must have been a major resource for the Ancestral Puebloans.

Excavated ruins of Antelope House in Canyon de Chelly revealed arrow mainshafts, dice, prayer sticks, basket fragments, a woven cradle back, and even cigarette fragments made from common reed. (We know this because some of the reeds were found with tobacco still inside.) In the course of excavating Aztec Ruins, numerous reedstem cigarettes were found, and at Chaco, prehistoric inhabitants had access to enough reeds to put a thick layer over the beams in some of the rooms.

Hopi have used common reed for roofing, pipe stems, weaving rods, and flutes. Ute once used the hollow stems to make composite arrow mainshafts, with a piece of sharpened, hard wood inserted in the tip as a point, and also for their red rock pipes. They strengthened the outside of their wickiups with reed and made floormats for the inside.

As far as we know, the Navajo were the only Four Corners people that used common reed for medicinal purposes. When taken as a mild emetic, the plant is said to have properties for curing stomach and skin problems. Common reed still grows in patches near most of the Rio Grande pueblos.

MARIPOSA LILY, SEGO LILY

Lily family
(*Calochortus gunnisonii, C. nuttallii*)

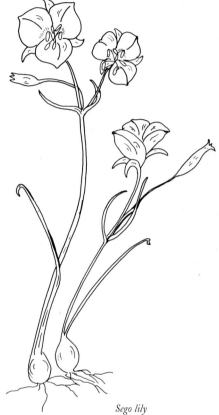

Sego lily

Like all lilies, mariposa lily floral parts (*C. gunnisonii*) come in threes: three petals, three sepals, six stamens, and three-lobed fruit. Petals are usually purple, although they can be white to yellow. Blossoms, which appear in early summer, are at the end of long, graceful stems, singly or in clusters of two or three. Mariposa lilies are found in mountain meadows and clearings in the piñon-juniper, ponderosa, and mixed conifer zones. They may occasionally be seen in shrubby areas on Chapin Mesa and elsewhere at Mesa Verde, as well as at Canyon de Chelly.

The very similar but shorter sego lily (*C. nuttallii*) usually has white petals, although they are known to come in purple and yellow. This is an early-blooming plant of the semi-desert and is especially abundant in Utah, where it occurs in large, fairly dense stands in sagebrush-covered flats, valleys, foothills, and open ponderosa parks at 4,500 to 8,000 feet elevation. Look for sego lilies at Mesa Verde, Hovenweep, and Canyon de Chelly.

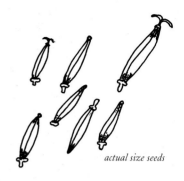

actual size seeds

All species of *Calochortus* have a gland of contrasting color at the inside base of each petal, and the leaves are grasslike. Before flowers appear, the leaves could be confused with those of the death camas (*Zygadenus* spp.), which has poisonous bulbs. The sego lily may be distinguished by the round, troughlike cross section of its U-shaped leaves as opposed to the V-shaped leaf of death camas. A sure way to tell the difference between the two is to wait until flowers appear; the clusters of small white death camas blooms have no resemblance to those of *Calochortus*.

Navajo and Hopi dig the bulbs of mariposa and sego lilies in early spring before they bloom. The bulbs are peeled and eaten raw or baked. These lilies are eagerly sought by children because the bulbs are very sweet.

Ute and Southern Paiute Indians used to dig sego lily bulbs in July and eat them immediately or bake them in an earthen oven. The seeds were ground for meal and the flower buds eaten raw.

Bulbs from both species are among the many wild plants that constitute Navajo Life Medicines. These plants are gathered and dried with other Life Medicine species and are usually saved for emergency situations. Four Life Medicine plants may be ground and mixed with water and drunk or rubbed on the skin, depending on the ailment, but it is said that it is better to have six or more mixed together (Mayes and Lucy 1989).

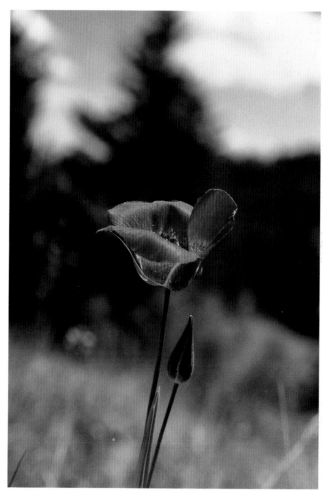

Mariposa lily

Sego lilies also figure prominently in Mormon history as a survival food that sustained the people when faced with famine conditions during drought and locust plagues. The sego lily is now honored as the state flower of Utah.

Buckwheat family
(*Eriogonum* spp.)

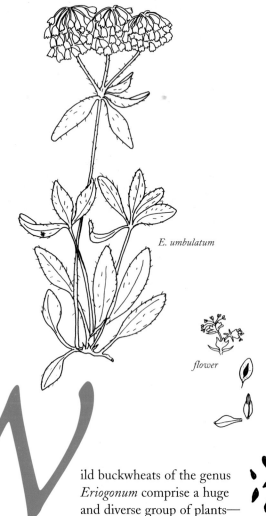

E. umbulatum

flower

Wild buckwheats of the genus *Eriogonum* comprise a huge and diverse group of plants—forty-one species grow in New Mexico alone and more than fifty in Utah. To the untrained eye there are no simple characteristics that define the buckwheats, although many of them can be recognized by slender branches that fork in pairs. The various-colored flowers for most species are papery and often form globular clusters.

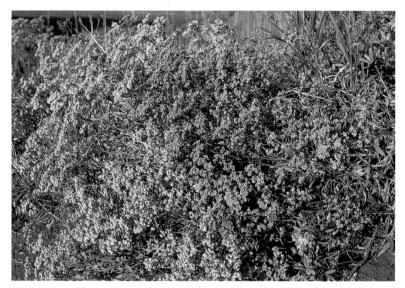

Eriogonum corymbosum

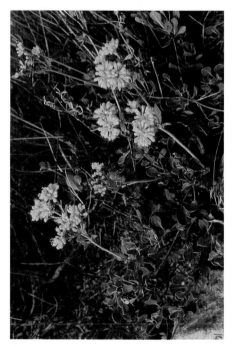

Sulfur buckwheat

Prehistoric remains of wild buckwheat are usually identifiable down to genus only. Two colorful species growing at Mesa Verde today, both with known uses from the past, are illustrated. One or more species of wild buckwheat may be found in all of the parks covered in this book.

The very word buckwheat conjures up images of pancakes or other flour-based foods. We don't know how the seeds of wild buckwheat were prepared in prehistoric times, but we do know they were being eaten as at least minor components of the Ancestral Puebloan diet at most sites where plant use has been analyzed, including those at Chaco and Mesa Verde. Carbonized wild buckwheat seeds have been recovered from a food storage vessel at one site in Arizona. There is a dearth of references to these plants as dietary items among contemporary peoples who have occupied the Four Corners area. One of the few references we were able to find is some sixty years old and relates to *E. corymbosum*, the shrubby wild buckwheat illustrated in our photo. "Among the Hopi the leaves are boiled, and with some water in which they are boiled they are rubbed on the mealing stone with corn meal, then baked into a type of bread" (Castetter 1935).

Medicinal uses for wild buckwheat abound in our region, however. The Hopi associate one or more species with medicine for menstruation and for expediting childbirth, as well as for relieving hip and back pain experienced by pregnant women. Ute Indians once used one species as a medicine, but little else is known about it.

Of course, the Navajo, who surely are the greatest practitioners of wild plant medicine in the Four Corners today, know of endless cures and healing powers for these plants. One species alone, redroot wild buckwheat (*E. racemosum*), "is used for a variety of internal injuries: blood poisoning, backache, sideache, venereal disease, and undefined internal injuries. The medicine is made by soaking the whole plant in water; the resulting liquid is drunk, or, for venereal disease, used as a lotion for sores" (Mayes and Lacy 1989).

Several species, including the illustrated sulfur buckwheat (*E. umbellatum*), are Navajo Life Medicines. Their plant parts are eaten as an emetic to cleanse the patient before a ceremony. Other medicinal applications of various species include a poultice of chewed leaves for ant bites, an infusion of whole plants for colds, and root extracts for diarrhea, sore gums, or contraception. One subtribe of the Navajo, the Ramah who reside in west-central New Mexico, recognizes and has separate medicinal uses for eight different species of wild buckwheat (Vestal 1952).

AMARANTH

Amaranth family
(*Amaranthus* spp.)

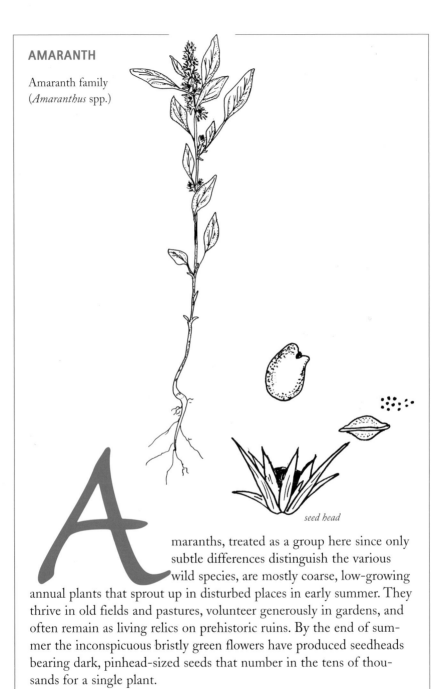

seed head

amaranths, treated as a group here since only subtle differences distinguish the various wild species, are mostly coarse, low-growing annual plants that sprout up in disturbed places in early summer. They thrive in old fields and pastures, volunteer generously in gardens, and often remain as living relics on prehistoric ruins. By the end of summer the inconspicuous bristly green flowers have produced seedheads bearing dark, pinhead-sized seeds that number in the tens of thousands for a single plant.

Each year the appearance of amaranths is a hit-or-miss proposition, depending upon spring and summer rains. They may occur in disturbed areas in any of the parks covered in this book.

Because amaranth seeds show up so consistently among plant remains examined at excavated archaeological sites throughout the Southwest, it is easy to speculate that weedy amaranths (also known as pigweeds) and their close cousins, the goosefoots (*Chenopodium* spp.), grew in abundance on human-disturbed land that would have been adjacent to most every Ancestral Puebloan village when it was occupied. Southwestern archaeobotanist Mollie Toll suggests that young, tender pigweed and goosefoot plants would have been collected by the ancient people and cooked as greens in late spring, while the seeds would be harvested toward the end of the growing season and probably parched prior to storage or grinding. Amaranth seeds were recovered beneath an overturned quartzite metate during the excavation of Salmon Ruin east of Farmington, New Mexico, and a quantity of black amaranth seeds was found stored in a bag at another Ancestral Puebloan site in the vicinity of Durango, Colorado. Indeed, amaranth seeds comprise a significant part of the food assemblage recovered from nearly every Ancestral Puebloan site that has been investigated in the Four Corners area.

The ancient people would not have known it, of course, but amaranth seeds are an especially good source of protein, containing more of the essential amino acid, lysine, than most true cereal crops. The greens are a healthy food, too, being rich in vitamins A and C plus iron and calcium.

As a group, amaranths are among the world's oldest crop plants, having been grown in the New World for more than two thousand years, although evidence is lacking for prehistoric cultivation of amaranths in the Southwest. However, plant remains dating to A.D. 100 or earlier from a once-inhabited shelter in south-central New Mexico, six hundred years later from a small pueblo in Chaco Canyon, and in present-day communities of native peoples attest to the long span of economic use of these plants.

Within the twentieth century, both seeds and greens of wild amaranth plants have been harvested by Hopi and Navajo. The latter thresh and grind the seeds into gruel to be eaten with goat's milk, or chew a handful of parched seed meal for a quick pick-me-up. Ute

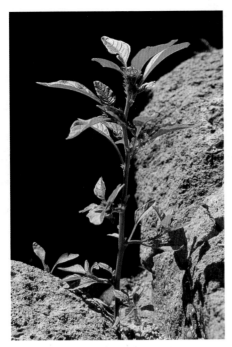
Wild amaranth

Indians used to collect seeds in autumn, grinding them into flour for cakes or mush. Southern Paiutes also once consumed both seeds and greens. The single recorded instance of amaranth cultivation in the Four Corners region during historic times comes to us from Dr. Edward Palmer, a contemporary of famed western explorer John Wesley Powell. Dr. Palmer reported in 1878 that the Paiute Indians were growing two different species of amaranth in their fields (Bye 1972). Unplanned cultivation is another matter, for amaranth "weeds" are not only tolerated but encouraged in many contemporary "old-style" Pueblo Indian gardens in the northern Rio Grande district.

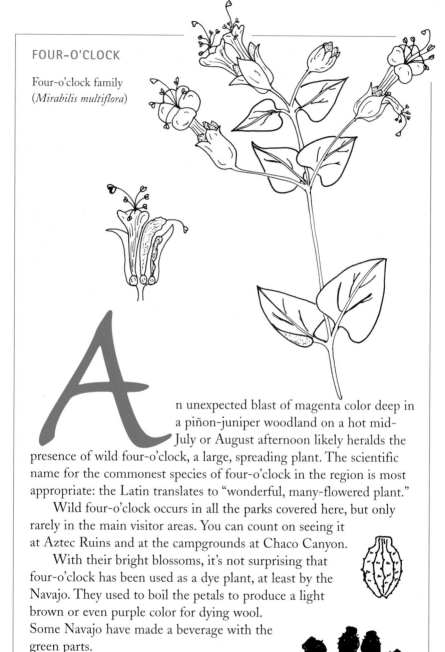

FOUR-O'CLOCK

Four-o'clock family
(*Mirabilis multiflora*)

An unexpected blast of magenta color deep in a piñon-juniper woodland on a hot mid-July or August afternoon likely heralds the presence of wild four-o'clock, a large, spreading plant. The scientific name for the commonest species of four-o'clock in the region is most appropriate: the Latin translates to "wonderful, many-flowered plant."

Wild four-o'clock occurs in all the parks covered here, but only rarely in the main visitor areas. You can count on seeing it at Aztec Ruins and at the campgrounds at Chaco Canyon.

With their bright blossoms, it's not surprising that four-o'clock has been used as a dye plant, at least by the Navajo. They used to boil the petals to produce a light brown or even purple color for dying wool. Some Navajo have made a beverage with the green parts.

But by far the most common use of this plant among groups of Indians inhabiting the

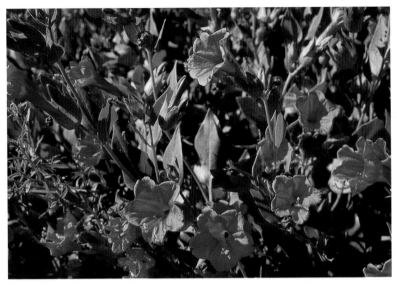

Four-o'clock

Four Corners has been medicinal. A long-lived perennial, older specimens grow a huge, thick root with cream-colored, almost crystalline pith, which is sought out for a variety of ailments. As recently as the mid-1970s, the root was being collected by Hopi and used as a blood strengthener for pregnant women. In Navajoland the ground boiled root has been used to treat mouth sores, rheumatism, and inflammation. Pueblo people seem to have discovered the most diverse pharmacological uses, including treatment for colic in babies, eye infections, muscle soreness, body swellings, rheumatism, and even indigestion. While the medicinal effectiveness of four-o'clocks is well known by most Indian groups in the region, it seems that no two groups share identical uses.

With all this traditional medicine, you'd think that wild four-o'clock plant parts would show up often in the archaeological record. They probably do, but the roots of this plant, which would most likely have been used, are not easily traced to *Mirabilis*. The closest record to the Four Corners area, one going back to hunter-gatherers of Archaic Indian time, comes from Fresnal Shelter, far to the south in New Mexico's Sacramento Mountains. From the large quantities of pulverized four-o'clock roots recovered here, it was concluded that they were being eaten at least two thousand years ago (Bohrer 1975).

PURSLANE

Purslane family
(*Portulaca* spp.)

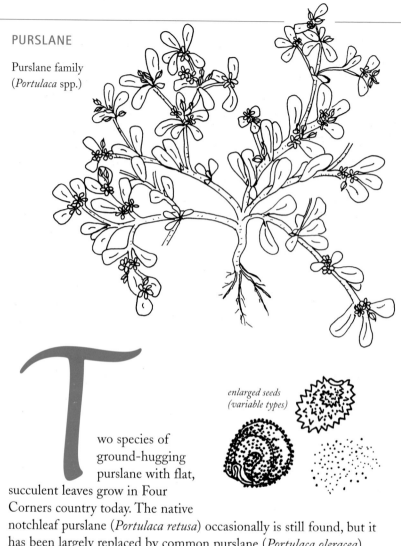

*enlarged seeds
(variable types)*

Two species of
ground-hugging
purslane with flat,
succulent leaves grow in Four
Corners country today. The native
notchleaf purslane (*Portulaca retusa*) occasionally is still found, but it
has been largely replaced by common purslane (*Portulaca oleracea*),
introduced into this country well over a century ago from Europe.
These annual weedy plants with minute yellow flowers that bloom
before midday pop out on bare ground almost anywhere below eight
thousand feet elevation where the soil has been disturbed and perhaps
lightly nourished by human activity. It may be encountered at any of
the parks covered herein.

Most gardeners in the Southwest recognize purslane instantly —
and promptly dispatch it with a weeding fork. Not so in times past,

for purslane was one of the most important wild plant foods for the Ancestral Puebloans and probably for their predecessors as well. Shiny black purslane seeds have been recovered from prehistoric hearths and from beneath a quartzite metate at Salmon Ruin on the San Juan River. They routinely turn up in coprolites at Chaco Canyon, Mesa Verde, and Canyon de Chelly and almost every other Ancestral Puebloan site that has been analyzed for ancient food consumption.

We can speculate that purslane would have thrived in and around ancient villages and fields wherever the soil was disturbed by human activity. It's likely that the green plant parts were prized at least as much as the seeds. These plants appear a little later in the season than the also-relished weedy amaranths and goosefoots and would remain palatable for many weeks after the others had grown too coarse for good eating. Great quantities of plants, those that were not stewed up immediately as greens, must have been basket-dried on pueblo rooftops away from rodents. The seeds could be stored separately and the dried leaves and stems saved for meals during winter.

Purslane would have been an excellent health food for the people because its parts are high in vitamins A and C and several B vitamins, as well as calcium, iron, and protein. Such a combination surely provided a good balance to the staple diet of corn and squash.

One of the earliest ethnobotanical records for the Southwest comes from renowned archaeologist J. Walter Fewkes who, in 1896, reported that the Hopi Indians boiled purslane leaves with meat. Navajo people made mush and bread from purslane seeds and also boiled or stewed the greens (Fewkes 1896). People from virtually all the Pueblo Indian nations have harvested this plant, as have probably every other group of Native Americans living in the Four Corners region. Fried in olive oil or butter, young purslane stems and leaves have a pleasant, mild flavor that is just a little on the sour side due to small quantities of oxalic acid stored there.

Purslane has been used medicinally by the Navajo for curing stomachaches and by Pueblo Indians as an antiseptic wash or as a treatment for diarrhea. Early texts that have been translated from the Maya Indians living in the Yucatán reveal that common purslane was eaten as a cure for consumption. If "a man shall fall ... or if he spits blood or if he vomits blood, take one handful of the *Portulaca oleracea*, its leaf and stalk together with its root. Boil this down to the quantity

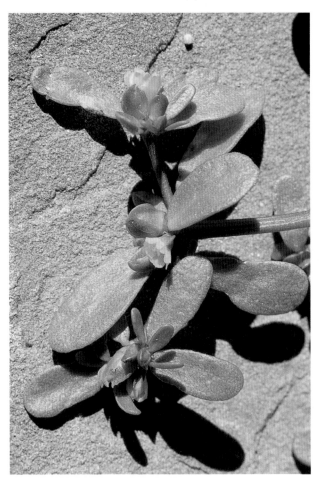
Common purslane

of a third of a drachm of honey, let it cool, add sufficient sugar to sweeten it and then give it to drink at dawn before breakfast for three or four days" (Roys 1931).

PRINCE'S PLUME

Mustard family
(*Stanleya pinnata*)

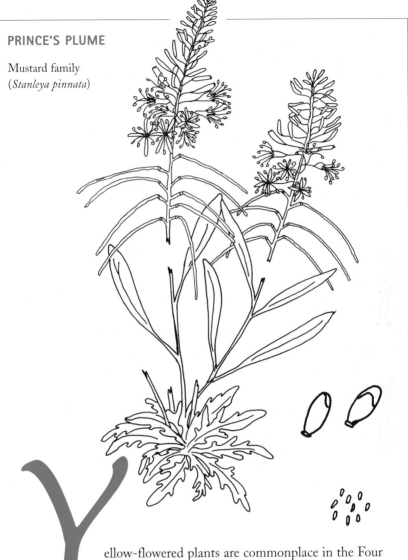

Y ellow-flowered plants are commonplace in the Four Corners region, but few have an elongated cluster of blossoms at the top of a two- to three-foot spindly stalk like this one. With four petals and six stamens, each prince's plume flower is typical of all plants in the mustard family. Long, narrow upper leaves and thin pods hang from the stalk below the flowers. These leaves and pods are frequently chewed off by animals; such is the case for this Chaco Canyon plant pictured on the next page.

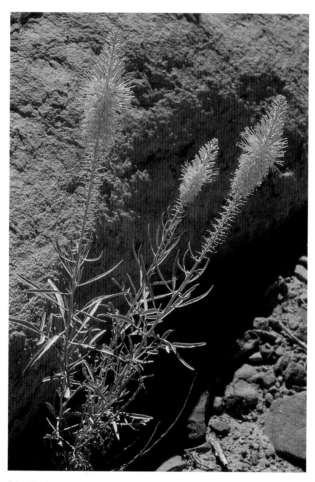

Prince's plume

Although never very common, these plants grow on dry plains in the desert shrub zone up to the lower slopes and mesas of piñon-juniper woodlands wherever the soil has a high selenium content. Look for prince's plume just above the canyon rim along the trail to Pueblo Alto at Chaco and in the vicinity of Balcony House at Mesa Verde. They also grow in a few places at Hovenweep, but not at Canyon de Chelly or Aztec Ruins.

We know of no records indicating Ancestral Puebloan use of this plant, but that is not surprising since it was the leaves that were cooked and eaten by Indians during historic times. In an archaeological context, green plant matter quickly disappears.

Tender leaves were collected by Hopi and Navajo for the table in spring, but they were always boiled before being eaten. These plants take up selenium from the soil where they grow, and selenium is poisonous to humans. Apparently, boiling removes most of the toxin if the water is discarded. The greens are usually boiled a second time.

Both greens and seeds have been a plant food for the Southern Paiutes. Until the end of the nineteenth century, the group living north of the Grand Canyon was almost entirely dependent on foods obtained in the wild. Isabel Kelly, who studied these people before they lost their land in this region, writes of prince's plume leaves being "… gathered in spring; boiled; drained; boiled again. Poured on grass to cool. Squeezed into small balls with hands…. Now cooked in frying pan with grease" (Kelly 1964).

As is the case for so many wild plants, the Navajo have some medicinal uses for *Stanleya*. For them it is one of their many Life Medicines. Prince's plume (probably raw) is used as an emetic and to treat glandular swellings. The cooked leaves taste like cabbage, so these plants were called wild-cabbage by early Mormon settlers.

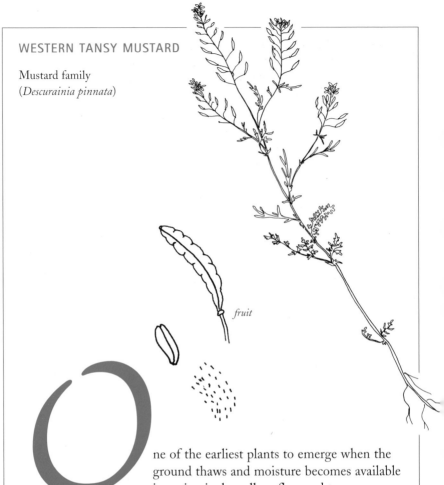

WESTERN TANSY MUSTARD

Mustard family
(*Descurainia pinnata*)

fruit

One of the earliest plants to emerge when the ground thaws and moisture becomes available in spring is the yellow-flowered tansy mustard. It prefers open land found along roadsides, in old fields and clearings and overgrazed pasture lands, and especially around prehistoric ruins.

Several species grow in the Four Corners region. Perhaps the commonest is *Descurainia sophia*, a weed introduced from Europe, which is recognized by its one-inch-plus, wire-thin fruits encasing minuscule seeds. Of much greater interest is the Western tansy mustard, which has fatter, half-inch-long seedpods and is native to the Four Corners region. This is one of several annual weedy plants, including amaranths and purslanes, that pops up in wet years on disturbed ground such as often surrounds ruin sites. Look for them along

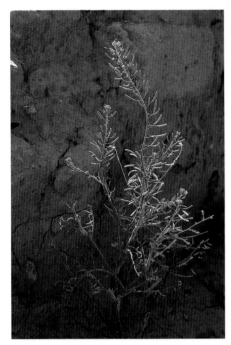
Western tansy mustard

the various trails on the valley floor and in the campground at Chaco Canyon and along the ruins loop roads at Mesa Verde. Only the introduced species grows at Aztec Ruins today.

Long ago tansy mustards were life-giving to the Ancestral Puebloans and basket-making people before them. Desiccated human feces that have been analyzed from archaeological sites regularly contain tiny red-brown tansy mustard seeds. In fact, seeds from this plant were among those found beneath a quartzite metate, a stone seed-grinding basin, at Salmon Ruin, a northern outlier of Chaco, and two gallons of such seeds once were collected from a much older burned-out ruin near Aztec, New Mexico.

If we consider Indian uses of tansy mustard in historic times, we can surmise that the greens were an important source of food for the ancients. Young plants that broke ground in profusion as early as March surely provided a welcome contrast, as well as nutritional balance, to the dried foodstuff of the long winter.

Southern Paiute people once cooked the greens as pot herbs and ground the seeds into flour for mush and bread. The Hopi still collect young tansy mustard leaves and cook them alone or add the salty-flavored greens to meat and vegetables; other Pueblo Indians also have harvested the iron-rich greens. The Navajo used to grind the seeds to make cake dough and other foods; those living near Kayenta, Arizona, once used a lotion made from plant parts to treat sore throats.

Because its leaves have a high iron content, tansy mustard ranks second only to beeplant (see page TK) for making soft-black to reddish paint for decorating pottery. Hopi and other Pueblo Indians living along the Rio Grande in New Mexico today boil the leaves and stems down to a gummy paste that may be wrapped in a corn husk and left to harden, similar to *guaco* (the pigment prepared from beeplant parts). The guaco cake is diluted with water and applied to a finished pot with a fine brush made of yucca fiber. Upon firing, this pigment takes on a brownish to light gray or gray-black hue. The Hopi tradition of using wild plant–based pottery paint is believed to have been carried down from Ancestral Puebloan times.

PEPPERGRASS

Mustard family
(*Lepidium* spp.)

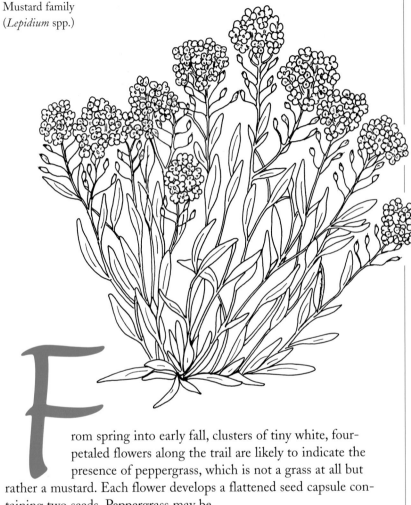

From spring into early fall, clusters of tiny white, four-petaled flowers along the trail are likely to indicate the presence of peppergrass, which is not a grass at all but rather a mustard. Each flower develops a flattened seed capsule containing two seeds. Peppergrass may be seen in all of the parks covered in this book except for Chaco Culture and Aztec Ruins, and it is prevalent along the main park road leading to the Mesa Verde visitor center.

fruit

capsules

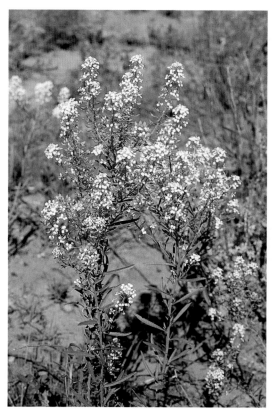
Peppergrass (*L. montanum*)

A single peppergrass plant may bear hundreds of seedpod fruits, and since the plants are ubiquitous throughout the Southwest, it is not surprising that the seeds were a staple in the Ancestral Puebloans' diet. Proof of this is found in studies of coprolites that have been analyzed from ruins at many sites in the Four Corners region. For example, from Antelope House at Canyon de Chelly National Monument, a recent study revealed the major components of coprolites dating around A.D. 1300 contained (in descending order of frequency) corn, amaranth seed, cactus epidermis, squash, horsebrush stem, cotton seed, peppergrass seed, Indian rice-grass seed, bean epidermis, pine nuts, purslane seed, and threeleaf sumac seed.

Peppergrass seeds are not particularly high in protein or total calories, but they are an excellent source of potassium, and the greens, which undoubtedly also were eaten, are rich in vitamin A.

The collection of peppergrass seeds for the table seems to have been abandoned early in historic times; the only reference to it in our area is one relating to the Southern Paiute Indians in the 1870s (Bye

1972). More recent medicinal uses were practiced at Isleta Pueblo south of Albuquerque, where it was reported that "The seeds are chewed as a relief for headaches" (Jones 1931), and from the Kayenta Navajo, who have employed plant parts to cure dizziness and gastrointestinal disorders. Navajo living around Chaco Canyon used peppergrass as a disinfectant.

Far to the south in the Yucatán of southern Mexico and Guatemala, an ancient text from the Mayans prescribes the seeds of *Lepidium medium* as a remedy for flatulence, and, in translation, the text states that "the crushed leaves are poulticed on swollen knees, itching pustules and wounds, and cuts" (Roys 1931). Sometime after the Spaniards' arrival, Mayans were reported to have concocted a beverage of ground peppergrass roots mixed with the introduced aloe to combat colds and coughs.

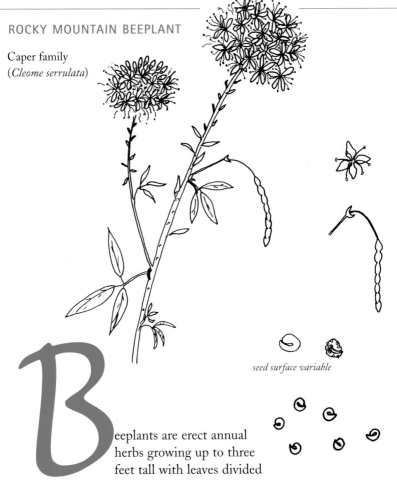

ROCKY MOUNTAIN BEEPLANT

Caper family
(*Cleome serrulata*)

seed surface variable

Beeplants are erect annual herbs growing up to three feet tall with leaves divided into spreading separate leaflets, delicate four-petaled flowers at the top of the stem and end of the branchlets, and long, often drooping, fruit pods. Lavender-flowered Rocky Mountain beeplant, the commonest species in our region, has leaves with three leaflets, while the leaf segments of the less familiar yellow beeplant (*C. lutea*) come in fives or more and the flowers, obviously, are yellow.

Rocky Mountain beeplant occurs sporadically on disturbed soil at Chaco and Canyon de Chelly; both species are rare at Mesa Verde and Hovenweep.

Coprolite evidence from Ancestral Puebloan remains at Chaco, Salmon Ruin, Mesa Verde, Canyon de Chelly, and other sites in the

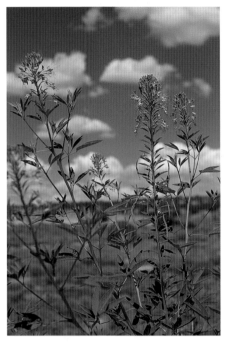
Rocky Mountain beeplant

Four Corners region indicates that beeplant seeds and probably greens were a regular part of the prehistoric diet. Since beeplant leaves are a good source of calcium and vitamin A, inclusion in the diet would have provided significant nutritional benefits. The frequency of beeplant pollen in packrat middens dating to 1000 B.C. at Canyon de Chelly, where the plant is not common today, suggests that people living in Archaic times may have encouraged this plant to grow around their dwelling places (Betancourt and Davis 1984).

Cleome thrives on disturbed ground, especially where the soil has been tilled, thus its other common name—*beeweed*. Large quantities of its pollen in combination with that of corn and squash have been identified from coprolites. This evidence suggests that beeplant was a leading foodstuff and that it was probably encouraged or even semi-cultivated in ancient fields.

The practice of encouraging *Cleome* in cornfields has been continued by the Hopi, who harvest and boil young plants with green corn. The Navajo also collect beeplant for the table. They prepare the greens like spinach, mix them with onions and meat in a stew, or grind up the seeds with salted ripe Indian corn and bake the dough into bread. According to Ute Indians, yellow beeplant greens also are edible.

As they have done with so many different wild plants, Navajo Indians have discovered medicinal uses for this group. Yellow beeplant has been associated with treating ant bites, and Rocky Mountain beeplant with ceremonial use. The Navajo make a shoe or moccasin deodorant from beeplant leaves soaked in water. Santa Clara Puebloans once used the leaves to treat stomach problems.

Navajo also create a yellow-green wool dye from beeplant. "The plant is picked before it flowers and boiled until tender. Next, the cooked plant is mashed, added to a pot containing yarn, and the mixture is allowed to ferment for a week. The yarn is allowed to ferment another week before being rinsed and dried" (Mayes and Lacy 1989).

Perhaps the most distinctive use of this plant was manufacturing black paint for pottery, baskets, and other objects from at least late Ancestral Puebloan times to the present. A concentrate of boiled leaves, called *guaco*, is dried and formed into little bricks. Pieces of guaco are mixed with water and applied like paint as a design to a pot after it is slipped and polished but before it is fired. Firing softens the black color to a dark gray.

LUPINE

Pea family
(*Lupinus* spp.)

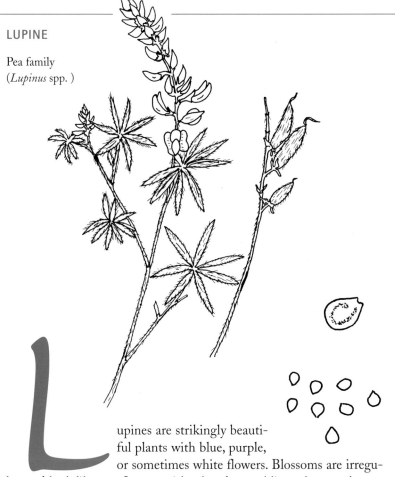

Lupines are strikingly beautiful plants with blue, purple, or sometimes white flowers. Blossoms are irregular, and look like pea flowers with a hood resembling a bonnet, hence the common name, "blue bonnet," in Texas. Numerous one- to two-foot-high stems produce flowers along the upper portions. Leaves are typically in five to fifteen leaflets, which resemble the palm and fingers of a hand. Foliage of all the southwestern species is slightly silvery with fine hairs. Seeds are borne in flattened pods that usually show a constriction between each bean. At maturity, the pods divide into two spiral pieces. Many species of lupine occur in our area, but they look so much alike that we won't distinguish them here.

Most lupines bloom profusely in early summer, then sporadically afterward. Commonly found in valleys in the piñon-juniper and ponderosa pine zones, they also thrive in historic fields and on roadsides,

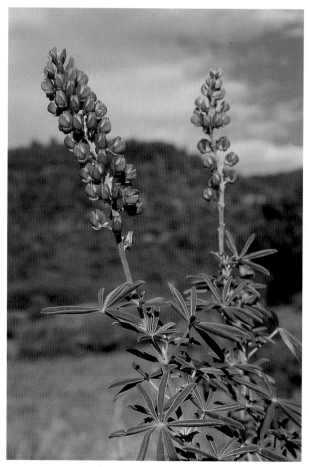

Spurred lupine

often in the poorest of soils. Lupines may occasionally be seen growing at Chaco and Canyon de Chelly. The most spectacular display we
found was at Mesa Verde's Morefield Campground, where spurred
lupine (*L. caudatus*) brightens the meadows in late summer.

There is no indication of lupine use from prehistoric sites, but
modern literature refers to contemporary use. Navajo boil the entire
plant, that is, flowers, leaves, and stems, with native alum (as a mordant) to make a greenish-yellow dye.

Both Hopi and Navajo use various species of lupine medicinally for external maladies. Because lupines are poisonous, they were not taken internally. The Hopi are said to make an eyewash from the plant, but no recipe is given. Navajo once ground the peeled roots into a paste that was applied to bruises, boils, and poison ivy blisters. They considered certain plant parts a remedy for sterility and to favor the siring of female children. Kayenta Navajo used the plant to cure ear-aches and nosebleeds and once planted ground leaves with watermelon seeds to ensure a good crop.

Lupines have been domesticated prehistorically in both the Old and New World. The plants are grown for fodder and to improve a soil's nitrogen content. Throughout the Mediterranean region and in South America, they have been selected for the large, white, edible seeds, but the processing of such seeds requires large quantities of fresh or running water. The seeds are washed in water and then allowed to soak in fresh water for three or four days. After soaking, they are cooked and rinsed again under running water. Finally, the seeds are dried and eaten as nuts that are rich in protein and edible oil.

No wonder the Ancestral Puebloans didn't use this plant for food; processing lupine beans to make them edible would have been nearly impossible in the arid Four Corners. Surely the people sampled wild lupine seeds and discovered they are bitter and cause a burning sensation in the mouth following the first taste, a warning that the seeds are poisonous. Spurred lupine, one of the most common species in our area, contains not only the poisonous compound lupinine but also a steroid that can affect growing embryonic cells and cause malformations of the fetus. Lupines are also poisonous to sheep, but are less so for horses and cattle.

BLAZING STAR

Loasa family
(*Mentzelia* spp.)

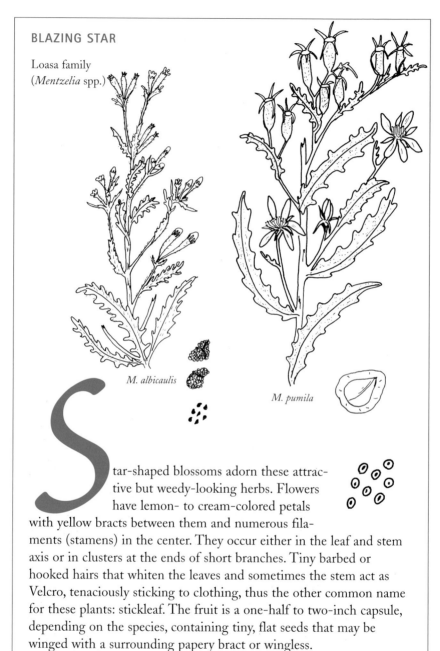

M. albicaulis

M. pumila

Star-shaped blossoms adorn these attractive but weedy-looking herbs. Flowers have lemon- to cream-colored petals with yellow bracts between them and numerous filaments (stamens) in the center. They occur either in the leaf and stem axis or in clusters at the ends of short branches. Tiny barbed or hooked hairs that whiten the leaves and sometimes the stem act as Velcro, tenaciously sticking to clothing, thus the other common name for these plants: stickleaf. The fruit is a one-half to two-inch capsule, depending on the species, containing tiny, flat seeds that may be winged with a surrounding papery bract or wingless.

Blazing star blooms from June through August. We have seen it in Chaco Canyon at the Gallo Campground, in the Ute Mountain

Ute Tribal Park, and along roadsides at Mesa Verde and on the Jicarilla Apache Reservation. Common stickleaf, *M. pumila*, also grows at Hovenweep and Canyon de Chelly.

On a kiva bench at Una Vida ruin in Chaco Canyon, archaeologists found an intact seed jar filled with unburned seeds of whitestem blazing star (*M. albicaulis*), the species most often associated with prehistoric sites (see page 74). Of all the species, it has the smallest fruit capsules and is one of very few species that does not have winged seeds. By all appearances, blazing star is another of the prehistoric annual weeds sensitive to available soil moisture. In years with significant precipitation, it was abundant; in years marked by less rain and snowfall, fewer plants grew. At Salmon Ruin seeds were recovered in prehistoric middens, thus were considered cultural artifacts.

In 1896 it was reported that whitestem blazing star seed was gathered by young Hopi women, then parched and ground into a fine sweet meal, served in a wicker basket, and eaten in pinches (Fewkes 1896). Based on plant collections made by Edward Palmer and John Wesley Powell in the 1870s, the seeds were also an important food for Southern Paiute Indians (Bye 1972).

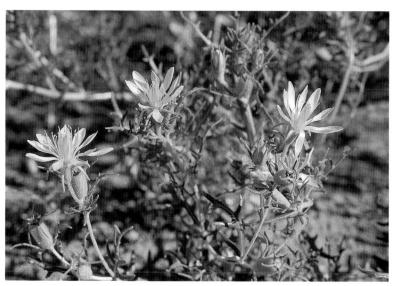

Common stickleaf

Seeds of both species were eaten by the Navajo, who also used blazing star as a medicine by putting parched, ground seed on small-pox sores to keep them from pitting. They may have realized that the sooner a wound scabs and the sooner the scab comes off, the less intense the permanent scaring. Common stickleaf is one of the many ingredients for Navajo Life Medicine. Rio Grande Pueblos as well as Hopi also had medicinal and ceremonial purposes for the plant.

Mentzelia is a New World genus. Most of its species are from Mexico and South America, and only a few are found in the American Southwest.

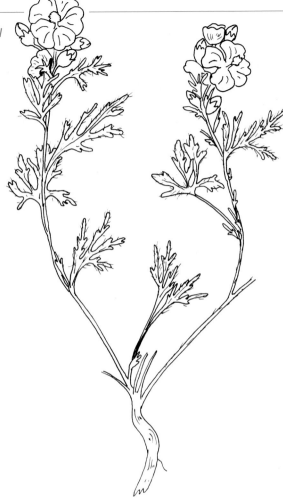

GLOBE-MALLOW

Mallow family
(*Sphaeralcea* spp.)

fruit

Several species of globe-mallow inhabit
open-space land in the Four Corners region.
They are especially common along road-
sides. All have distinctive blossoms resembling miniature
hollyhocks, with a central pollen-bearing column surrounded
by five petals—usually orange or red-orange, but some
varieties pink or violet. Tiny star-shaped tufts of hair
cover the foliage.

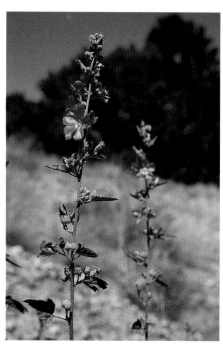

Scarlet globe-mallow (*S. coccinea*)

The giveaway orange flowers are commonly seen throughout the summer on the floor of Chaco Canyon and at Aztec Ruins. Globe-mallow is less common at Mesa Verde, while a pink-flowered species occasionally grows at Canyon de Chelly along with the orange ones.

Globe-mallow seeds and flower parts turn up regularly in the plant remains examined at prehistoric sites from Mesa Verde and the Colorado Plateau to Chaco Canyon and south into Rio Grande country. Clearly, the compressed globular fruits and probably other plant parts were eaten by the ancients, but was it for their food value or for medicinal purposes? At Chaco, prehistoric globe-mallow pollen grains are more often associated with the inside of kivas than with food preparation rooms. Furthermore, use by Indians in this region during historic times is nearly always medicinal, although long ago globe-mallow was said to be eaten by Navajos and Puebloans during the leanest of times.

In our area, medical applications of globe-mallow during the past century are legion. Rio Grande Puebloans have applied ground roots to snakebites and sores to draw out venom and to stem inflammation. The Hopi used a paste made from the ground roots to cast broken bones. (The same property made it useful in hardening adobe floors.) They also combined ground roots with cholla fruits to create a mixture used to treat diarrhea.

The Navajo word for globe-mallow translates to "medicine that covers." Thus, Navajo have used a liquid mix of roots to arrest bleeding and as a lotion for skin disease. According to *The Purpose and Uses of Plants of Navajoland* curriculum manual recently published by the Chinle Curriculum Center near Canyon de Chelly, "Globe-mallow is used as medicine to treat stomachaches much as Pepto-Bismol is used as a home remedy." Indeed, one species of globe-mallow, *Sphaeralcea coccinea*, is one of the Navajo's Life Medicines and is employed as a tonic to improve appetites and to cure coughs and colds. The Navajo are also known to have dried the leaves and used them for tobacco.

The stiff-haired leaves have been rubbed on sore muscles at certain northern Pueblos or ground up to treat rheumatism at others. Ute Mountain Ute people used to pound the leaves and rub the smashed vegetal matter on infections, including acne.

PRICKLY PEAR

Cactus family
(*Opuntia phaeacantha*,
polyacantha and similar species)

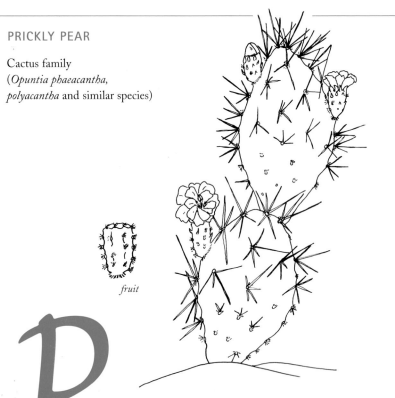

fruit

Prickly pear cacti are easily recognized by their flat, stout-spined stems arranged in a jointed series of pads. Several species grow in Four Corners country. Some are erect with juicy pads covered with relatively few spines (*O. phaeacantha*); others have a prostrate growth form, densely spined pads, and rather dry pads and fruits (*O. polyacantha* or *erinacea*). The flowers of most prickly pears are yellow. One or more of these cacti occurs at all the parks covered in this book except Aztec Ruins.

The fruits were regular dietary items for most Ancestral Puebloans, although at Chaco, where the fleshy-fruited species is absent today, they seem to have played a minor role. Much farther south, the Aztecs of Mexico recognized thirteen varieties of prickly pear fruits, some sour, some sweet; some were eaten raw, others were cooked. The ancient Maya Indians also ate them (Coe 1994). Prickly pear *tunas*, as the fruits are known, would have provided a good source of protein, vitamin C, potassium, and calcium.

In more recent times prickly pear has been recorded as a food item for Hopi, Rio Grande Pueblo, Navajo, and Southern Paiute Indians. Navajo tell of removing the spines by rolling the fruit in sand or singeing them in hot ashes.

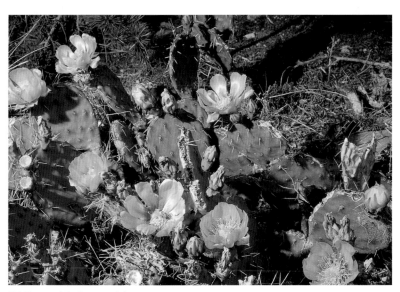

Ripe red tunas are still one of the most important wild plant dye sources for traditional Navajo rug weavers. The women steep their wool yarn for days or weeks in a solution of water and unboiled, fermented tuna juice to produce various hues of rose and pink. Different shades can be created by adding toward the end of the dyeing process root bark from mountain-mahogany or other plants. Ute Indians sometimes used cactus juice to temper their pots before firing.

Marilyn Colyer, longtime resource management chief at Mesa Verde National Park, has observed that in recent years a high percentage of prickly pear fruits in the Mesa Verde region are devoid of seeds and therefore are sterile. She wonders whether this is the result of a natural genetic change since the time when the seeds were so plentiful in Ancestral Puebloan diets or whether pollution or another form of human interference accounts for this condition.

Prickly pear (*O. phaeacantha*)

HEDGEHOG CACTUS

Cactus family
(*Echinocereus* spp.)

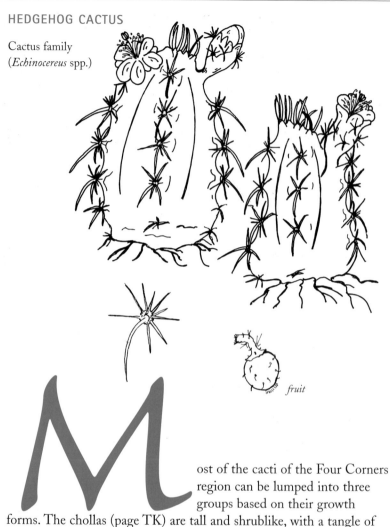

fruit

Most of the cacti of the Four Corners region can be lumped into three groups based on their growth forms. The chollas (page TK) are tall and shrublike, with a tangle of jointed cylindrical stems; prickly pear stems are flattened and padlike; while the hedgehog and pincushion cacti are low-growing with oval or columnar-shaped single or multiple stems. All of these, of course, bear spines.

The stems of all hedgehog cacti are ribbed. Most of the species in the Four Corners have flowers ranging from pink to deep red. Look for these cacti growing on rimrock at Mesa Verde, Hovenweep, and Canyon de Chelly but not at Chaco.

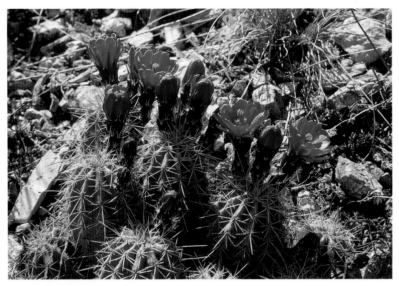

Claret-cup cactus

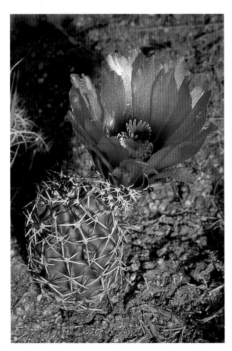

Fendler hedgehog

Fleshy, thin-skinned hedgehog cactus fruits are considered someof the tastiest among the several groups of cacti. Although they are smaller than prickly pear fruits, their flavor is sweeter, and as the fruits mature, the spines loosen and thus are more easily removed. Evidence from a number of archaeological sites, including Chaco and Salmon Ruin, confirms that fruits were collected and eaten during early Ancestral Puebloan times. The Hopi continue to relish the fruits of one species, Fendler hedgehog (*E. fendleri*), collecting them in spring, then drying them 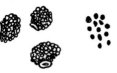 for later use as a food sweetener. Other Pueblo Indians living along the Rio Grande in New Mexico sought out the fruits of another hedgehog, claret-cup cactus (*E. triglochidiatus*), for preserving.

It's likely that all the other tribes that have lived in Four Corners country enjoyed hedgehog cactus fruits; indeed, food use has been reported across the Navajo Nation and among the Southern Paiute living in Utah. The thick, juicy stems of these cacti and those of the pincushion cactus group (*Coryphantha* and *Mammillaria* spp.), which tend to be smaller and usually have a single stem, undoubtedly would have served as food for various tribes in times of famine.

The only medicinal record we have for these cacti is from Isleta Pueblo, located south of Albuquerque. At one time Isletans roasted the stems of one species and put them on sores to reduce swelling.

EVENING-PRIMROSE

Evening-primrose family
(*Oenothera* spp.)

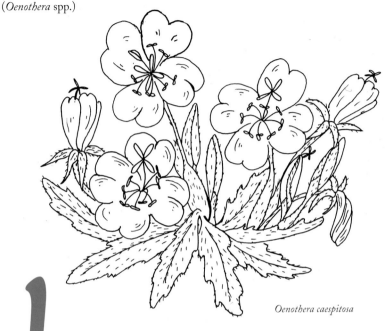

Oenothera caespitosa

I n the Four Corners region the many species of evening-primrose can be *annuals*, blossoming from seed each year; *biennials*, sending out a rosette of leaves the first year and blooming the second; or *perennials*, longer-lived and blooming every year. Charming, fragrant flowers are white to pink or yellow and one to three inches across. When listening carefully, one can actually hear them pop open in the late afternoon or early evening. All primroses have four petals and a cross-shaped stigma in the center of the flower. They grow at elevations ranging from 4,000 to 8,500 feet. Most *Oenothera* are from the temperate New World. Some of the yellow-flowered species appear to be adapted to natural meadows or abandoned historic fields.

While in season, which is most of the early summer, the ubiquitous evening-primrose lines roadsides and dots broad arroyo bottoms.

A locally popular name for one of the white-flowered species is Kleenex plant, and landowners have been known to hop out of their cars in rage to clean up the tissue waste someone carelessly threw out, only to find that the offending material was an evening-primrose blossom. We have seen the whitish-flowered plants along the roadsides to Mesa Verde and Chaco Canyon and the tall yellow ones at Aztec and Mesa Verde. They also occur at Hovenweep and Canyon de Chelly.

Although the genus *Oenothera* is native only to the New World, by the mid-1600s one or more species had been introduced from North America to Europe, where they were cultivated for their edible leaves, roots, and shoots. Indigenous people of the Four Corners have eaten them for a long time also, but the prehistoric record in the Southwest is practically nonexistent. We know of only one reference, and that is from *Oenothera* seed found in a ruin at Chaco Canyon. Being uncharred, this seed may have been introduced by rodents, and

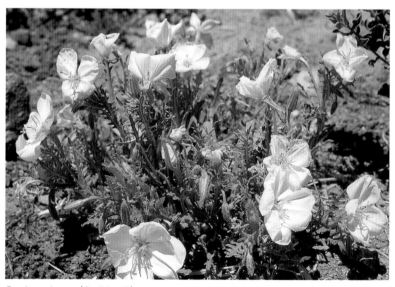

Evening-primrose (*O. albicaulis*)

the ethnobotanist who identified it is uncertain of its prehistoric, if any, connection.

The Hopi smoked *Oenothera albicaulis* as a tobacco and used another species to ward off the common cold. They also treated sore eyes with evening-primrose parts and associate the white flowers with the northeast direction.

Navajo utilize many different species for medicine; in fact, several are included in their Life Medicine mix. In the form of a liniment, evening-primrose has been used for treating boils. Roots were ground to treat stomachaches and the flowers mashed and applied as a dusting powder on sores or as a poultice for spider bites. Mixed with flax and wild buckwheat, it was a remedy for kidney disease. A hot poultice made with the yellow-flowered *O. hookeri* mixed with white clay and corn pollen was applied to sores and swollen glands resulting from mumps and was used for colds, perhaps as a throat or chest plaster.

Navajo living in the vicinity of Canyon de Chelly once used evening-primrose for gynecological problems, specifically a prolapsed uterus. Certainly the native people of the Four Corners region were onto something in the medicinal application of these plants. Recently, oil of evening-primrose has been shown to be effective in treating feminine disorders and is now a common natural remedy found in all modern health food stores.

SACRED DATURA

Tomato family
(*Datura meteloides*)

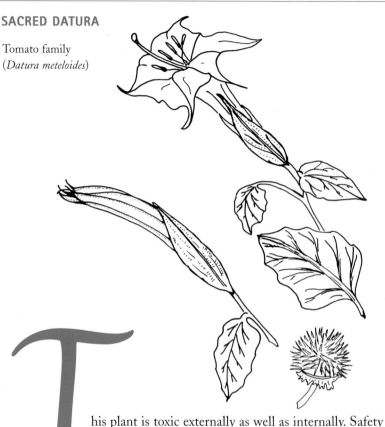

This plant is toxic externally as well as internally. Safety dictates that you *not touch it!* Looking every bit like a fugitive from the tropics, this lush, sprawling mound of a plant is found where a little bit of extra water makes suitable habitat for plants and a haven for people in an inhospitable land. The white-to-violet-colored flowers resemble huge lilies, and they emit a heavy, sweetish fragrance. Stems and foliage are thick and usually covered with fine hairs that sometimes give them a gray cast. Fruits are round and spiny. This is a sturdy perennial, and, once established, the roots of older plants can become huge, sometimes weighing twenty pounds or more. Some see sensuality in the appearance of this plant, others something sinister.

There are only about twenty species of datura in the world, and most are found in the American Southwest and in Mexico. Sacred datura or western jimsonweed, Indian-apple, or *tolache*, as it is called in the borderlands, grows in sandy washes, disturbed sites, grottos, and sometimes near roadsides. We have found it at Hovenweep and along the bottom of Canyon de Chelly; it also occurs at Chaco, but not Mesa Verde.

Its distribution is so disjunct—that is, plant populations are few and very far between—that some ethnobotanists and archaeologists believe the principal method of dispersal may have been by direct or indirect human action. And, as another member of the solanaceous plant complex discussed in chapter 8, it may have been introduced from Mexico in ancient times along with medicinal prescriptions for its use. Seeds and pollen have been found throughout the prehistoric Greater Pueblo area, but no modern use has been reported from any of the eastern pueblos along the Rio Grande. However, all the western pueblos are reported to have used it on occasion.

Sacred datura is a hallucinogen, a potent narcotic, and a medicine of magnificent potential when used by a trained medicine person. In

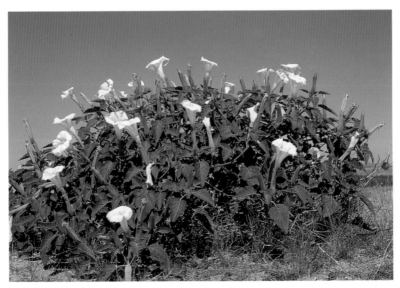

Sacred datura

excessive doses, it can cause death or permanent insanity; twenty seeds can kill a man. Used responsibly, as reported by Zuni, Kayenta Navajo, and other southwestern tribes, it is a powerful analgesic that can be used effectively to deaden pain when fractured bones are set, ulcerated wounds are cleansed, and during simple operations. The Hopi and Navajo are aware of sacred datura's toxic quality; for this reason they fear and avoid the plant. Nevertheless, and not too long ago, medicine men have made use of it.

An early report (Castetter 1935) describes the Navajo using fruits of sacred datura as food. They ground the fruit with a special kind of clay and ate it plain or dried. They stored the large capsules for winter, at which time they were soaked, boiled until tender, and then ground with this clay before eating. The clay probably neutralized the toxicity, but Castetter's description of the preparation suggests that the heat created by grinding or boiling also may have dissipated some of the alkaloids. Considering that even the plant's fragrance can make one nauseous or lull children into a drugged sleep, it would take a lot of neutralizing for us to try it. We recommend that you see this plant for its beauty and historic significance but leave it untouched.

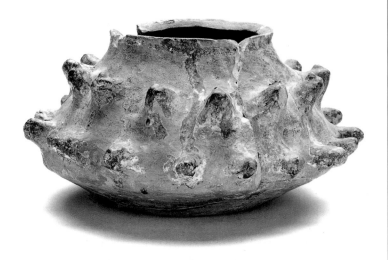

Ceramic jar, Pueblo culture ca. A.D. 1515–1620, apparently modeled after sacred datura fruit.

SCARLET PENSTEMON

Snapdragon family
(*Penstemon barbatus*)

SKYROCKET

Phlox family
(*Ipomopsis aggregata*)

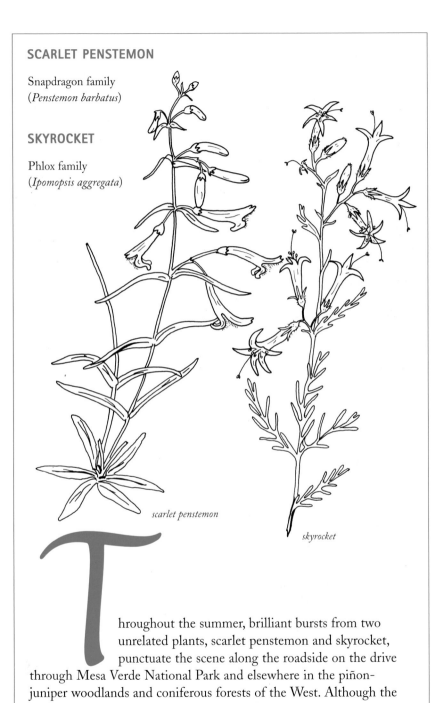

scarlet penstemon

skyrocket

hroughout the summer, brilliant bursts from two
unrelated plants, scarlet penstemon and skyrocket,
punctuate the scene along the roadside on the drive
through Mesa Verde National Park and elsewhere in the piñon-
juniper woodlands and coniferous forests of the West. Although the

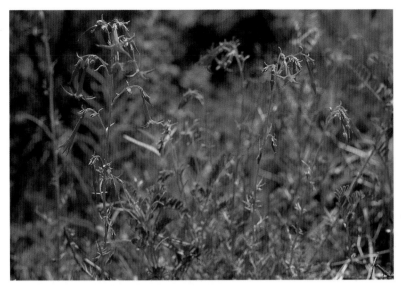

Skyrocket

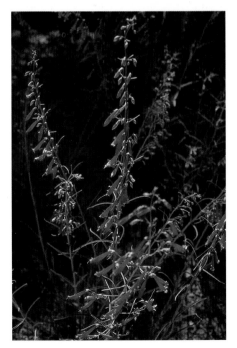

Scarlet penstemon

color and size of their flowers are nearly identical, the two species can be easily differentiated. Scarlet penstemon has narrow, tubular, snapdragon-shaped blooms about one-and-a-half inches long, and its leaves are narrow. At one to three feet tall, the slightly shorter skyrocket (also known as scarlet gilia) has trumpet-shaped flowers bearing floral tubes that expand into five pointed lobes at the tip and leaves that are finely divided.

At Mesa Verde, scarlet penstemon is especially common along the trail to

Spruce Tree House, where earlier in the season another close relative, the red-flowered Eaton penstemon (*P. eatonii*), could be confused with it. The latter plant is distinguished by its wider paired leaves that have crinkled edges and seem to clasp each stem. Skyrocket and scarlet penstemon occur infrequently in the other parks covered here; they are not nearly so attention-getting as at Mesa Verde.

Both are medicine plants, especially for the Navajo. Scarlet penstemon is one of their many Life Medicine plants, that is, it is collected and used in combination with parts from other wild plants to effect healing. Extracts from the roots of this penstemon are associated with treating arrow and gunshot wounds, as well as relieving menstrual pain, coughs, stomachaches, and burns. Although several other species of penstemon grow in Navajoland and are associated with medicinal cures, this one seems to be the most highly valued. Navajo used to boil scarlet penstemon flowers to concoct a sweet drink.

It is skyrocket's leaves that provide the medicine. At one time dried skyrocket leaves were stirred in water and drunk by the Navajo as a general remedy for stomach problems. For both the Navajo and the Hopi, a leaf extract has been swallowed to help ensure good luck in hunting. Hopi women also may drink a boiled skyrocket-leaf mixture shortly after giving birth.

THISTLE

Sunflower family
(*Cirsium* spp.)

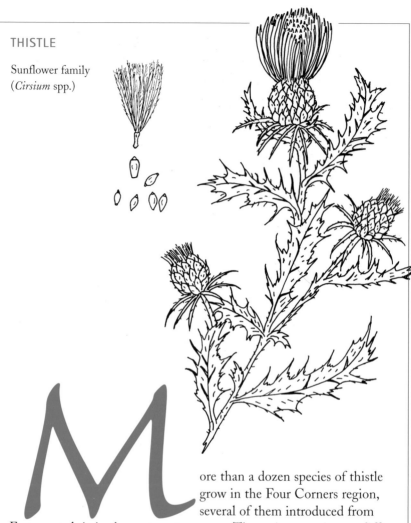

More than a dozen species of thistle grow in the Four Corners region, several of them introduced from Europe or Asia in the past century or so. The various species are difficult to tell apart in the field, so we treat them all as generic thistles.

As a group, thistles are easily recognized from their tall growthform, prickly leaves, and large, compact flower heads, each resembling a rose-colored powder puff (although some species are yellow or white). Many of the thistles, especially those that were introduced, thrive along roadsides and other waste ground. They are fairly common in disturbed places throughout Mesa Verde and in the campground at Chaco but less so at the other parks covered in this book.

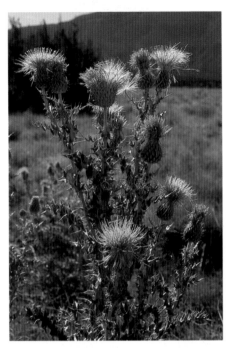

Thistle (*C. ochrocentrum*)

Charred thistle remains, indicating human use, have been recovered from a very few Ancestral Puebloan sites, but how the plants fit into the prehistoric scheme of things is unknown. It seems likely that thistles were much less common in this region before the introduction of several species in historic times.

The only regional reference we have on the food use of thistles indicates the Southern Paiute Indians once ate its stems. However, throughout the Great Basin north and west of the Four Corners, the stalks of several different thistle species were regular food items, prepared by peeling the prickly outer skins and consuming only the inner pith.

Medicine is another matter. The Hopi once drank tea from thistle plant parts to cure colds and relieve constipation. Rio Grande Puebloans from San Juan Pueblo applied thistle seeds to skin boils, and Zuni Puebloans formerly considered a tea made from crushed roots to be an effective contraceptive.

Thistles are one of the Life Medicine ingredients for the Navajo, who usually do not distinguish between the various species. The most consistently applied medicinal practice seems to be for treating various eye problems. A cold infusion of the root may be administered as an eyewash for sore or swollen eyes. Combating fevers and headaches are other Navajo uses.

During our visit to the Ute Mountain Tribal Park, we were told that thistle flower heads once were used by Ute people as a sort of toothbrush, although we never did determine exactly how this was accomplished.

ROCK GOLDENROD

Sunflower family
(*Solidago petradoria*)

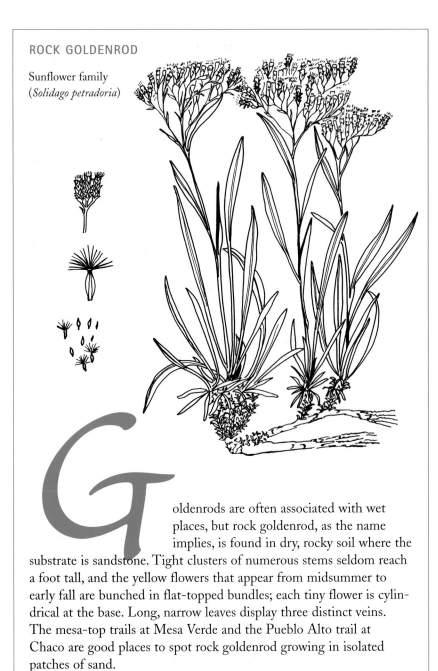

Goldenrods are often associated with wet places, but rock goldenrod, as the name implies, is found in dry, rocky soil where the substrate is sandstone. Tight clusters of numerous stems seldom reach a foot tall, and the yellow flowers that appear from midsummer to early fall are bunched in flat-topped bundles; each tiny flower is cylindrical at the base. Long, narrow leaves display three distinct veins. The mesa-top trails at Mesa Verde and the Pueblo Alto trail at Chaco are good places to spot rock goldenrod growing in isolated patches of sand.

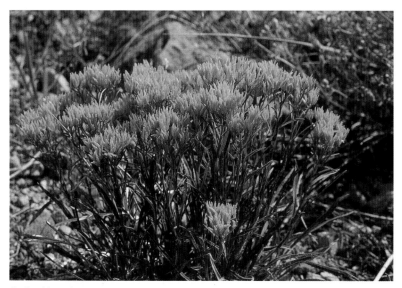
Rock goldenrod

Plant parts from rock goldenrod have been used by Hopi women to decrease the flow of breast milk and to alleviate chest pains. The leaves may be cooked with corn for various other remedies. Navajo combine them with other wild plants to concoct a ceremonial beverage to purge the body and to bring about spiritual renewal. They also used rock goldenrod to treat ant bites (and even a swallowed ant) and to heal external injuries, since a cold infusion of the leaves acts as an astringent.

Although one species is native to Europe, *Solidago* is principally a North American genus and has been widely used across the continent for medicinal purposes. Several other species of goldenrod grow in our region, and their leaves have been used for food (Hopi), an emetic (Acoma and Laguna pueblos), and general pain relief (Zuni Pueblo). For some species it is the roots that are collected for healing purposes.

Goldenrod flowers are just one of several different yellow-petaled composites that have been used by the Hopi to produce a wide range of yellow and gold tones for dying cotton, wool, or baskets. Early Anglo settlers also used goldenrod blossoms for this purpose. Acoma Puebloans formerly collected stems from one of the riparian species of goldenrod for crafting rough baskets.

PURPLE ASTER

Sunflower family
(*Machaeranthera* spp.)

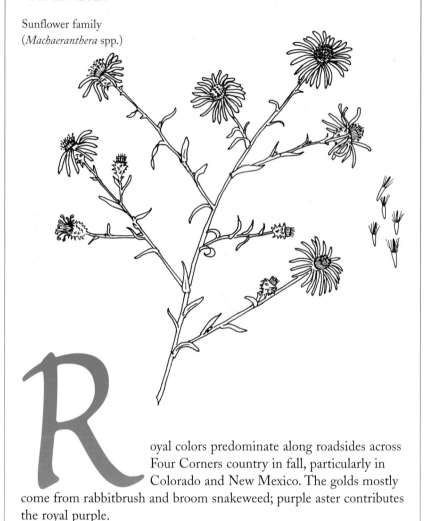

R oyal colors predominate along roadsides across
Four Corners country in fall, particularly in
Colorado and New Mexico. The golds mostly
come from rabbitbrush and broom snakeweed; purple aster contributes
the royal purple.

The many-branched, usually upright stems terminate in bluish to
purple (rarely white), asterlike flower heads that have yellow centers.
Leaves of most species have bristly tips or margins. One or more
species of purple aster occurs in or nearby all the parks covered in
this book.

Perhaps because ancient remains of so many of the hundreds of
species of sunflower family plants are difficult, if not impossible, to

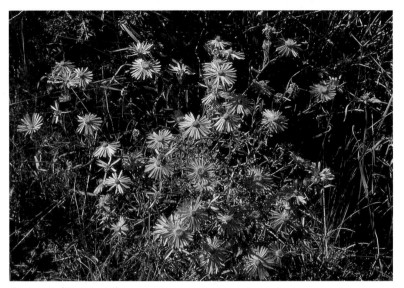
Purple aster (*M. tephrodes*)

distinguish, purple asters have not been recorded from any archaeological site context. However, the descendants of Ancestral Puebloans practiced several medicinal applications for plant parts.

The Hopi considered a concoction of leaves and stems to be a strong stimulant, especially effective for women in labor. In New Mexico, Zuni Puebloans drank a tea made from ground up plants as an emetic for an upset stomach. Along the Rio Grande, Puebloans chewed fresh blossoms to settle the stomach.

Navajo also have made an extract from the whole plants to treat stomachaches. Navajo from the Ramah area just east of Zuni dried and pulverized the roots of one purple aster, *Machaeranthera tanacetifolia*, and used it to cause sneezing in order to clear nose congestion.

You'd think the deep purple flowers of some purple asters would be an important ingredient for producing native dyes, but the record shows otherwise. The only dye use we have come across is from Acoma Pueblo, well south and east of the Four Corners, where the people once mixed ground purple aster petals with white clay to produce a dye for wool, but the color achieved probably was temporary.

Sunflower family
(*Senecio* spp.)

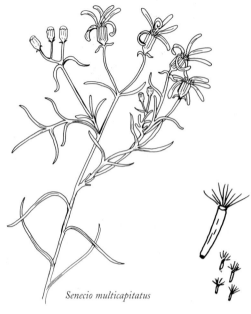

Senecio multicapitatus

Like so many other composites—a family of plants that comprises the largest number of plants in the Four Corners as well as in the rest of North America—groundsels, or butterweeds as they sometimes are called, are yellow-flowered. Plants in the genus *Senecio* are best recognized by the arrangement of the involucre, the series of green bracts that encloses the base of the flower heads. Groundsels have tightly packed, cylindrical involucres that resemble a miniature picket fence.

We won't differentiate the many kinds of groundsel here; more than fifty species grow in the Southwest (and 310 have been identified in South Africa). From late spring through fall various kinds of groundsel can be seen growing at Mesa Verde, Hovenweep, Chaco, and Canyon de Chelly.

Groundsels mainly have been used for medicinal purposes in the Four Corners region and throughout the world. Many of them contain senecionine, an alkaloid that has soothing effects when administered in the proper dosage.

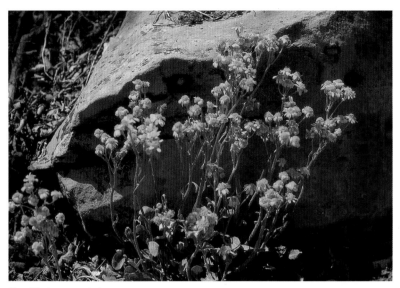
New Mexico groundsel

In the past, the Hopi pounded the leaves of two different species with a hot rock and smeared the paste over sore muscles. Ground leaves also were used by Hopi to treat pimples. Pueblo Indians from Zuni, New Mexico, have made eye drops from the blossoms of one of these species (*S. multicapitatus*), and Rio Grande Puebloans once made a tea from another, *S. douglasii*, to treat severe stomach trouble.

Navajo use groundsel in these same ways, but they also associate various species with many other treatments, including medicine for arthritis, rheumatism, and boils. A cold extract from the root of *S. multicapitatus* was used by the Ramah Navajo as an aid in childbirth. In times of famine, these people would collect and roast the seeds of this plant. Mixed with cornmeal and goat's milk, the result was a reasonably palatable gruel.

A cold extract of New Mexico groundsel, the species featured in the photograph, was said by some to bring good luck in hunting. This same plant has been smoked as tobacco in several ceremonies by Navajo living in the vicinity of Canyon de Chelly.

The alkaloids contained in some Four Corners species can cause irreparable liver damage. Thus, one must not experiment with groundsels.

INDIAN TEA

Sunflower family
(*Thelesperma megapotamicum*)

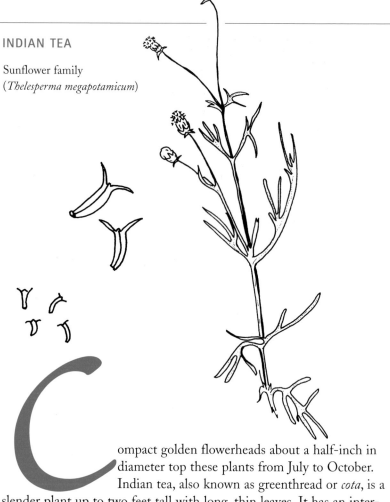

Compact golden flowerheads about a half-inch in diameter top these plants from July to October. Indian tea, also known as greenthread or *cota*, is a slender plant up to two feet tall with long, thin leaves. It has an interesting distribution, growing on open slopes, piñon-juniper mesas, and flats in the Rocky Mountain states from Wyoming to Mexico; then it skips over all the tropical countries and appears again in southern South America. You may find it at Chaco but not at Mesa Verde or Canyon de Chelly, where open, treeless land is scarce.

Indian tea is universally sought for brewing a hot beverage by people from all Indian tribes and quite a few Hispanics and Anglos who live in Four Corners country today. The consensus is that the slightly smoky-flavored beverage produced from *Thelesperma* is the best of the wild herb teas in our region. Felipe Lauriano, from Sandia

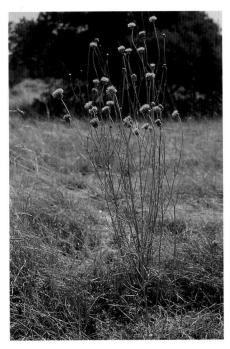
Indian tea

Pueblo just north of Albuquerque, told us how he and many others prepare it: "You can tie a bunch of stems and flowers with string and hang the bundle in your house to dry. Then in winter when it gets cold, you boil it just like Lipton's for a tea which has a dark red-orange color and tastes really good."

Something in this plant makes the tea act as a diuretic, and so it is considered a medicinal herb by the Navajo, who drink it for urinary problems. Like many other teas, it's supposed to be good for indigestion.

This is one of several wild plants used to produce shades of orange and gold dyes for cotton and wool fibers and baskets. The Hopi consider Indian tea the best of all plants for creating the richest, most permanent hues. They use a stronger infusion of flowers and stems than for making tea and vary the color and intensity by adding raw alum, smoking the dyed material, or soaking it in a solution of stale urine (for the effect of ammonia). The Hopi achieve a deep red-brown for their wicker or yucca baskets by placing the dyed item in a smoker for several hours. Navajo weavers may add other wild plants such as dock (*Rumex hymenosepalus*) or mountain-mahogany root bark (*Cercocarpus montanus*) to the wool dye mix to create different shades of orange. Traditional Jicarilla Apache basketmakers use Indian tea stems to produce a red-orange dye.

With such a variety of known uses for Indian tea during historic times, the Ancestral Puebloans also must have used the plant in some way, but positive evidence is lacking.

Sunflower family
(*Helianthus annuus*)

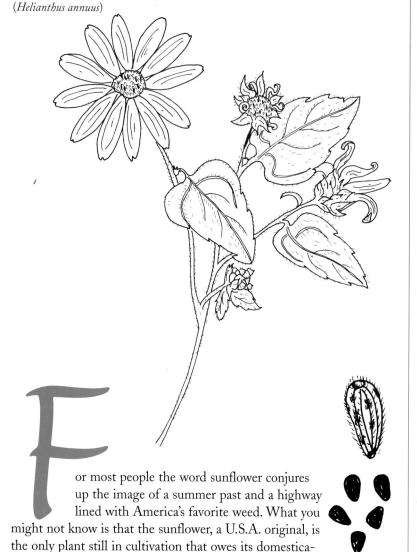

For most people the word sunflower conjures up the image of a summer past and a highway lined with America's favorite weed. What you might not know is that the sunflower, a U.S.A. original, is the only plant still in cultivation that owes its domestication to Indians who once occupied this country.

Sunflower heads are made up of individual golden outer flowers, called *straps* or *rays*, that encircle the tightly packed central brown disc

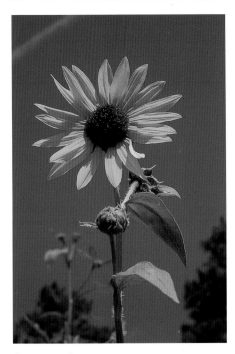
Common sunflower

flowers. Only the disc flowers develop into seed. Prairie sunflowers (*H. petiolaris*) are short, about knee-high, and spindly, with many small flowers; they share much the same habitat as the other species but blossom a little earlier. Common sunflowers (*H. annuus*) are tall, up to six feet or more, with a stout central stalk and fewer flowers at the ends of their many branches. You will find them growing along roadsides, in abandoned fields or vacant lots, and anyplace else in the Four Corners where the soil is regularly scratched up a bit and grass isn't competing for local nutrients.

Giant sunflower, the ten-foot-tall one that you see propped up on garden fences in rural towns, is a domesticated variety of the common sunflower. These have a single thick stalk topped with a giant flower head that can reach a foot in diameter and often needs support.

Years ago a southwestern archaeologist discovered thirty beautifully carved and painted wooden sunflowers in a large corrugated ancestral Puebloan pot. Murals incorporating painted sunflower designs were found on ancient Hopi kiva walls. At Chaco Canyon and Mesa Verde analyzed coprolites containing pieces of wild sunflower seed hulls confirm that these seeds were an important prehistoric food item.

The Hopi grow a particular variety of single-headed sunflower that is tall, slender with dark leaves, and has a thin, dark purple seed that requires a longer growing season to mature than other local varieties. This sunflower is prized for the brilliant blue, purple, black, or red dye that is made from the hulls and used to dye wool, cotton, and basketry. After the color has been removed, hulls are cracked and the meat of the seed eaten. The oily seeds are ground with corn to make a beverage called *pinole* or to grease the stone cooking griddle. Hopi still use a "spider medicine" made from prairie sunflowers.

Navajo mixed the seeds of cultivated sunflowers with corn, ground the mixture into a meal, and then shaped it into cakes to be baked. It seems likely that they obtained this particular sunflower variety from the Hopi since Navajo also boiled the outer seed coatings in the same manner to obtain a dull, dark-red dye. Navajo also attribute medicinal qualities to sunflowers, including a treatment for prenatal infection and another for removing warts. A cold extract of entire prairie sunflower plants is one of their many Life Medicine ingredients.

The sunflower itself is a splendid ecological niche—a whole world to tiny creatures. Some summer day take a look at a sunflower stalk and you will see that it hosts black ants, ladybugs, spiders, aphids, and numerous other miniature beasties, all very busily traveling about their tiny world of stalks and flowers.

ARROWLEAF BALSAMROOT

Sunflower family
(*Balsamorhiza sagittata*)

MULESEARS

(*Wyethia arizonica; W. scabra*)

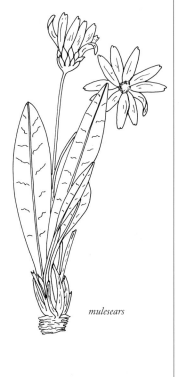

mulesears

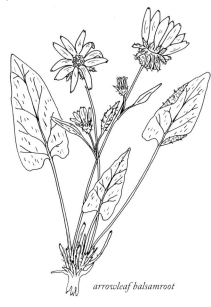

arrowleaf balsamroot

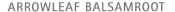

balsamroot seeds

T wo members of the sun-
flower family, each bearing
large yellow flowers, brighten
in early summer the roadsides leading to the
park museum and the ruins loop roads at Mesa Verde National Park.
Both grow up to two or more feet tall and are quite similar looking,
except that mulesears has long, aromatic, straplike leaves (thus the

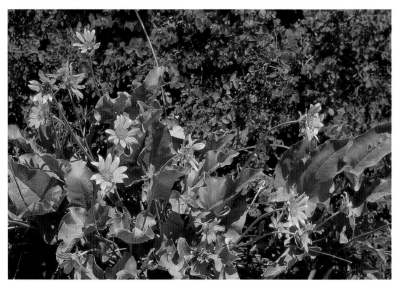
Arrowleaf balsamroot

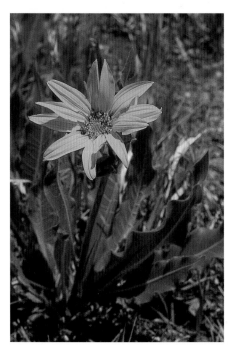
Mulesears

name), while arrowleaf balsamroot has equally long but distinctly arrow-shaped leaves. Both plants occur infrequently at Hovenweep National Monument, and mulesears may occasionally be spotted along the rim roads at Canyon de Chelly.

There is no record for either of these plants being collected for the household in prehistoric times (although it's likely that they were), and both rank as somewhat minor in importance for more recent use. However, they illustrate how two similar species growing in the same geo-

mulesears seeds

graphical region can be utilized very differently.

Arrowleaf balsamroot is mainly a food plant. Raw young shoots and leaves, and even the ample taproot, raw or cooked, were still being eaten around the turn of the century by Ute Indians. In the old days Southern Paiute Indians living in northern Arizona and southern Utah gathered balsamroot seeds from the higher plateaus in the fall and then roasted and ground them for flour.

The thick taproot of mulesears is also said to be edible when cooked, but more often this plant is used for making medicine. Navajo living in the vicinity of Canyon de Chelly found that parts of this plant act as an emetic and use it to treat stomachaches and heartburn. The Hopi ingested mulesears to cleanse the body, but "the use of this plant as an emetic is said to be dangerous, since if it is not removed from the stomach by vomiting, it will kill the patient" (Whiting 1939).

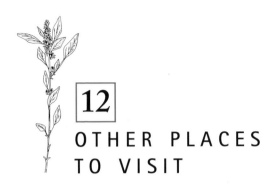

12
OTHER PLACES TO VISIT

S O FAR WE HAVE FOCUSED on five different parks where you will find the wild plants described in this book. But of course many other parks in the region have excellent interpretive trails, as well as museums that relate to our story of wild plants and their uses by native peoples. Some of these places are briefly described below. Included are parks that feature a combination of interpretive centers and walking trails, along with several public museums and centers that will be of interest to those who care to learn more about the subject. To help you obtain up-to-the-minute information, the address of each park or facility follows the description.

Museum of Indian Arts and Culture One of four museums in Santa Fe that is operated by the Museum of New Mexico, this museum is technically outside the Four Corners area but it surely has the most thorough coverage of our subject, displaying and interpreting a superb collection of prehistoric and recent Southwest Indian pottery and other artifacts. A major permanent exhibit added in 1997 tells the story of native peoples who have lived for twelve thousand years in the region covered in this book. Temporary displays and traveling exhibits often deal with native plant uses and related subjects. Bookstore features southwestern history, and an extensive library and archaeological and research collection are available for public use. Open daily except for major holidays; entrance fee. 708 Camino Lejo, Santa Fe, New Mexico 87504.

Salmon Ruin Museum and Heritage Park Salmon Ruin, on the banks of the San Juan River between Farmington and Bloomfield, New Mexico, was one of the larger outlier villages occupied by the people of the Chaco Canyon culture during the eleventh century. Besides the ruins themselves, facilities here, operated by the San Juan County Museum Association, include an interpretive trail that features the identification and ethnobotanical uses of wild plants, as well as a small museum. Open daily all year except for major holidays; modest entrance fee. P. O. Box 125, Bloomfield, New Mexico 87413.

Southern Ute Cultural Center and Museum The town of Ignacio in southern Colorado is headquarters for the Southern Ute Indian Tribe and is the location of this museum and Indian gift shop. Exhibits tell about the tribe based upon creation stories and the Ute point of view; the adjoining gift shop offers Ute beadwork, jewelry, and art from other Indian tribes. Open daily in summer with a restricted schedule in winter; modest entrance fee. P. O. Box 737, Ignacio, Colorado 81137.

Anasazi Heritage Center Located just eighteen miles by highway from Mesa Verde National Park, the Anasazi Heritage Center, operated by the Bureau of Land Management, emphasizes hands-on exhibits that involve kids and grown-ups alike. It takes a modern approach to teaching how Ancestral Puebloans who lived in the Four Corners region coped with their environment. Museum exhibits also explain techniques employed by modern archaeologists. A short self-guiding trail leads to a nearby ruin. Open daily except for major holidays;

modest fee. 27501 Highway 184, Dolores, Colorado 81323.

Crow Canyon Archaeological Center   This center is committed to building a greater understanding of Ancestral Puebloans who once occupied the Four Corners region. Located just northwest of Cortez, Colorado, the center serves throughout the year as a school for cultural exploration by many amateur and professional participants from all over the United States. In summer, hands-on day programs also are available by reservation for groups touring the region. Call (970) 565-8975 or write the center, 23390 County Road K, Cortez, Colorado 81321.

Ute Mountain Tribal Park   This park, just south of Mesa Verde and actually larger than that national park, has been set aside within their reservation by the Ute Mountain Ute Tribe to preserve Ancestral Puebloan culture. Here, cliff dwellings, surface ruins, historic Ute wall paintings, and ancient petroglyphs are surrounded by unbelievable scenery. Moderately priced full-day and half-day tours are offered by contacting the Tribal Park at (970) 565-3751 or by writing the park director c/o Towaoc, Colorado 81334.

Natural Bridges National Monument   Forty miles west of Blanding, Utah, on Highway 95, this unit of the National Park System preserves three of the world's greatest water-formed geologic arches. Although natural features are the focus of this park, you can also see and learn about the Ancestral Puebloan ruins found here. Open daily. Visitor center, campground, and many trails off the one-way loop drive. Box 1, Lake Powell, Utah 84533-0101.

Navajo National Monument   Twenty miles west of Kayenta, Arizona, off U.S. Highway 160, a paved road leads to Navajo National Monument, site of two of the largest and most dramatic prehistoric cave villages. Betatakin and Kiet Siel Ruins are among the best preserved in the Four Corners region. As descendants of the Ancestral Puebloans who lived there eight hundred or more years ago, several contemporary Hopi clans claim direct ties to these sites, and Hopi elders make an annual visit to pay respect. Trails, some easy, others very strenuous, lead to overlooks or to the ruins themselves. The Park includes a fine museum and a Park Service campground and picnic area. Open daily. HC-71, Box 3, Tonalea, Arizona 86044-9704.

Hopi Villages   The Hopi mesas and their villages are reached via Highway 264, which runs from Gallup, New Mexico, to Tuba City, Arizona. Several of the villages retain a classic Puebloan atmosphere, and Oraibi is regarded as the oldest continuously inhabited settlement in the United States. The visiting public is allowed in most places, but photography, recording, and sketching are strictly prohibited. Hopi craftsware are displayed and sold from many of the homes, and there also are craft centers, a small museum, and, at Second Mesa, a motel. Hopi dance ceremonies are held throughout the year, with many of them open to the public. Contact the Office of Public Relations, The Hopi Tribe, P.O. Box 123, Kykotsmovi, Arizona 86039, or telephone (602) 734-2441.

Museum of Northern Arizona   If you are anywhere near Flagstaff, a visit to this privately funded museum is a must, for it covers many of the subjects featured in this book, with room after room of first-rate displays. The bookstore is superior, carrying almost every title in print dealing with past and present Indian peoples of the Colorado Plateau. Open throughout the year; admission fee. 3001 North Fort Valley Road, Flagstaff, Arizona 86001.

Hubbell Trading Post National Historical Site   Also on the same highway that links the Hopi villages (Arizona Highway 264), Hubbell Trading Post, just outside Ganado, Arizona, is one of the oldest of the continuously operated posts on the Navajo Reservation. Visitors can get a sense of the past when Indian traders supplied many of the daily needs of Navajo people and the Navajo had a common place to display and sell their rugs, jewelry, and other crafts. Here one can purchase Navajo-crafted items, visit a Park Service museum, and attend various guided events, including craft demonstrations. Open all year. Box 150, Ganado, Arizona 86505.

Navajo Nation Museum   Just east of Window Rock, Arizona, on Highway 264, this free museum provides a good interpretation of Navajo Nation history, including the development of native arts and crafts. Next door the Navajo Arts and Crafts Center displays and sells traditional and contemporary rugs, jewelry, baskets, and other wares. Open Mondays through Fridays all year. Navajo Nation Historical Preservation Department, P.O. Box 9000, Window Rock, Arizona 86515.

Suggested Reading

Eddington, Patrick and Susan Makov
1995   *Trading Post Guidebook: Where to Find the Trading Posts, Galleries, Auctions, Artists, and Museums of the Four Corners Region.* Northland Publishing, Flagstaff.

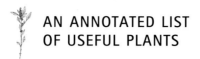

AN ANNOTATED LIST
OF USEFUL PLANTS

The following list of useful wild plants is a compilation of plants occurring in the Four Corners region that are known to have been used by native people occupying the region—either past or present. Nomenclature normally follows the authority of Martin and Hutchins 1980 or Kearney and Peoples 1960. The list is based on a comprehensive review of the technical literature as well as information collected personally by the authors. Domesticated or recently introduced plants and uses that are mainly ritualistic are not included.

The list covers flowering plants plus ferns and their allies; however, only four species of grasses are included. Numerous other useful grasses are principally those associated with obscure Navajo medicinal applications. A total of 515 useful species are included in the list that follows. In many cases (e.g. *Allium* (2), *Amaranthus* (4), etc.), only the genus is listed where the two or more useful species in that genus have similar uses. The number following a genus indicates the number of species used in the region. Listing all species would have exceeded available space.

Plant uses are subdivided into seven general categories. The native users in historical times are Hopi, Navajo, Ute, Jicarilla Apache, and Southern Paiute that have lived within the region. Prehistoric uses are derived from archaeological evidence, published or conveyed directly to the authors by contemporary authorities. The cited references comprise only a fraction of the literature that was consulted.

Key to Chart

USERS:

PH: prehistoric; **PH?** Prehistoric use uncertain (usually food or medicine); **HO:** Hopi; **NA:** Navajo; **UT:** Ute; **JI:** Jicarilla Apache; **SP:** Southern Paiute; **MO:** Universal use (historical).

REFERENCES:

1. two or more authorities; **2.** personal knowledge by authors of this book; **3.** Adams 1980a; **4.** Adovasio et al, 1986; **5.** Bryan and Young 1940; **6.** Bye 1972; **7.** Callaway et al, 1986; **8.** Castetter 1935; **9.** Chamberin 1909; **10.** Chinle Curriculum Center 1995; **11.** Colton 1965; **12.** Colton 1974; **13.** Doebley 1981; **14.** Elmore 1944; **15.** Fewkes 1896; **16.** Fowler 1986; **17.** Fry and Hall 1986; **18.** Hall and Dennis 1986; **19.** Kelly 1964; **20.** Hocking 1956; **21.** Jones and Fonner 1954; **22.** Magers 1986a; **23.** Magers 1986b; **24.** Mayes and Lacy 1989; **25.** Minnis and Ford 1977; **26.** Morris 1980; **27.** Nichols undated; **28.** Opler 1936; **29.** Peckham 1990; **30.** Pettit 1990; **31.** Smith 1974; **32.** Stiger 1977; **33.** Toll 1993; **34.** Vestal 1952; **35.** Wheeler 1994; **36.** Whiting 1939; **37.** Williams-Dean 1986; **38.** Windes and Ford 1996; **39.** Wyman and Harris 1941; **40.** Wyman and Harris 1951.

	FOOD, BEVERAGE, SMOKING	MEDICINE	CONSTRUCTION, FUEL	IMPLEMENTS, CEREMONIAL	BASKETS	TEXTILES, CORDAGE, MATTING	DYE, PAINT, TANNING, SOAP
Abies concolor (white fir)			PH 38				
Abronia fragrans (sand verbena)		NA, UT 1, 9					
Acer glabrum (Rocky Mountain maple)		NA 34					
Acer negundo (box-elder)				PH, NA 22, 14			
Achillea lanulosa (yarrow)		NA,UT,SP 1, 9, 6					
Adiantum capillus–veneris (maidenhair fern)		NA 40					
Agastache pallidiflora (giant hyssop)		NA 34					
Agoseris aurantiaca (mountain-dandelion)		NA 1					
Allionia incarnata (umbrellawort)		NA 34					
Allium spp. (2) (wild onion)	MO 1						
Alnus tenuifolia (alder)				PH 23			NA 1
Amaranthus spp. (4) (amaranth)	PH, MO 1, 1	NA 39					
Amelanchier spp. (2) (serviceberry)	PH,HO,NA,UT,SP 25,1,1,1,19	NA 1		PH,HO,UT,SP 1,36,1,19			
Ammannia coccinea (ammannia)	SP 6						
Amorpha sp. (false indigo)		NA 14					
Androsace spp. (3) (rock-jasmine)		NA 1					
Anemopsis californica (yerba mansa)	PH, SP 13, 6	NA 39					
Anthericum torreyi (crag lily)		NA 34					
Apocynum spp. (4) (dogbane)		NA 1				SP 6	
Aquilegia sp (columbine)		NA 40					
Arabis fendleri (Fendler rockcress)		NA 34					
Arctostaphylos spp. (3) (bearberry)	NA, SP 1, 1	NA, SP 1, 6					
Arenaria spp. (4) (sandwort)		HO, NA 36, 1					
Artemisia tridentata (big sagebrush)	PH? 32	MO 1	PH 1	PH, NA 23, 14	UT 31	UT 1	NA, SP 5,6
Artemisia spp. (6) (sagebrush)	HO, NA, SP 36, 1, 6	HO, NA, SP 1, 1, 6					

	FOOD, BEVERAGE, SMOKING	MEDICINE	CONSTRUCTION FUEL	IMPLEMENTS CEREMONIAL	BASKETS	TEXTILES, CORDAGE MATTING	DYE, PAINT, TANNING, SOAP
Asclepias spp. (2) (milkweed)	HO 15	HO, NA 36, 1					
Aster spp. (4) (aster)		NA 34					
Astragalus spp. (11) (milkvetch)	HO 15	NA 1					
Atriplex canescens (fourwing saltbush)	PH?, SP 1, 6	NA 1	PH, HO 1, 15	HO 36			HO, NA 36, 1
Atriplex concertifolia (shadscale)	PH, HO, SP 17, 15, 6						
Atriplex spp. (4) (saltbush)	PH?,HO,NA,SP 18,1,1,6	NA 34					NA 34
Baccharis spp. (2) (baccharis)		NA 1		NA 40			
Bahia spp. (3) (yellow ragweed)		NA 1					
Balsamorhiza sagittata (arrowleaf balsamroot)	UT, SP 9, 19						
Berberis spp. (2) (barberry)	SP 1	HO, NA 36, 1		PH, HO 26, 36			NA 1
Besseya plantaginea (kittentails)		NA 34					
Betula occidentalis (western water-birch)				PH 23			
Brickellia spp. (3) (brickelbush)		NA 1					
Calliandra humilis (false mesquite)		NA 34					
Calochortus spp. (2) (sego/Mariposa lily)	HO,NA,UT,SP 1, 1, 1, 1	NA 34					
Campanula parryi (Parry's bellflower)		NA 34					
Carex spp. (2) (sedge)		NA 34					
Castilleja spp. (4) (paintbrush)		HO, NA 36, 1					NA 5
Caulanthus crassicaulus (caulanthus)	SP 6						
Ceanothus fendleri (buckbrush)		NA 1					
Celtis reticulata (netleaf hackberry)	PH, NA 1,1						NA 14
Cercis occidentalis (western redbud)	NA 1						
Cercocarpus montanus (mountain-mahogany)		NA 1		PH,HO,NA,UT 1,12,1,7			HO, JI 11,2
Chamaesaracha coronopus (chamaesaracha)		NA 40					
Cheilanthes wootonii (lipfern)		NA 34					
Chenopodium spp. (7) (goosefoot)	PH,HO,NA,SP 1,1,1,6	NA 40		PH 22			

	FOOD, BEVERAGE, SMOKING	MEDICINE	CONSTRUCTION, FUEL	IMPLEMENTS, CEREMONIAL	BASKETS	TEXTILES, CORDAGE, MATTING	DYE, PAINT, TANNING, SOAP
Chrysothamnus spp. (3) (rabbitbrush)	NA 24	HO, NA 1,1	PH 33	PH, HO 27, 36			HO, NA, JI 1,1,2
Chrysopsis spp. (3) (golden aster)		NA 34					
Cicuta maculata (water hemlock)		NA 10					
Cirsium spp. (4) (thistle)	SP 16	HO, NA 36, 1					
Claytonia lanceolata (spring beauty)	SP 6						
Clematis spp. (2) (virgin's bower)		NA 1					
Cleome lutea (yellow beeplant)	UT 2						
Cleome serrulata (Rocky Mountain beeplant)	PH, MO 1,1			PH 23			PH, HO, NA 1, 1, 1
Coldenia hispidissima (coldenia)		NA 40					
Comandra pallida (bastard toadflax)	SP 6	NA, UT 1,9					
Commelina dianthifolia (dayflower)		NA 34					
Conioselinum scopulorum (hemlock-parsley)		NA 40					
Conopholis mexicana (Mexican squawroot)		NA 39					
Corallorhiza maculata (spotted coralroot)		NA 40					
Cordylanthus wrightii (Wright clubflower)		NA 1					
Coreopsis cardeminefolia (tickseed)		NA 34					
Corispermum sp. (bugseed)	PH? 1	NA 1					
Cornus stolonifera (red-osier dogwood)	SP 6	NA 1					
Corydalis aurea (golden corydalis)		NA 1					
Cosmos parviflora (cosmos)		NA 34					
Cowania stansburiana (cliffrose)		HO, NA 36, 1		HO 36		HO, NA, UT, SP 36, 1, 2, 1	NA 1
Croton texensis (doveweed)		HO, NA 36, 1					
Cryptantha spp. (5) (hiddenflower)	PH 1	HO, NA 1, 1					SP 6
Cucurbita foetidissima (buffalo gourd)		SP 6					SP 6
Cuscuta megalocarpa (dodder)		NA 34					
Cycloloma atriplicifolia (winged pigweed)	PH 1	HO 36					HO 36

	FOOD, BEVERAGE, SMOKING	MEDICINE	CONSTRUCTION FUEL	IMPLEMENTS CEREMONIAL	BASKETS	TEXTILES, CORDAGE, MATTING	DYE, PAINT, TANNING, SOAP
Cymopterus spp. (6) (wafer-parsnip)	MO 1	NA 1					
Datura meteloides (jimsonweed)		PH?,HO,NA,SP 23, 1, 1, 6					
Daucus pusillus (wild carrot)	NA 1						
Delphinium spp. (2) (larkspur)	HO 12	HO, NA 1, 14					NA 5
Descurainia pinnata (western tansy mustard)	HO, NA, SP 1, 34, 1	NA 40					PH, HO 29, 36
Descurainia sp. (tansy mustard)	PH 1						
Ditaxis cyanophylla (ditaxis)		NA 34					
Dithyrea wizlisenii (spectacle-pod)		HO, NA 1, 1					
Draba spp. (2) (whitlowgrass)		NA 1					
Dyssodia papposa (fetid marigold)		NA 34					
Echinocereus spp. (2) (hedgehog cactus)	PH,HO,NA,SP 1, 8, 8, 16						
Eleocharis spp. (2) (spikerush)		NA 34					
Ephedra spp. (2) (joint-fir)	PH?, NA, UT 1, 24, 2	MO 1					NA, JI 5, 2
Epilobium ciliatum (willowweed)		NA 40					
Equisetum spp. (3) (horsetail)	HO 15	NA 1					
Erigeron spp. (7) (fleabane)		NA 1					
Eriogonum corymbosum (wild buckwheat)	HO 8						
Eriogonum inflatum (desert trumpet)	SP 6	NA 40					
Eriogonum umbellatum (sulpur wild buckwheat)		NA 40					NA 5
Eriogonum spp. (7) (wild buckwheat)	PH? 1	HO, NA, UT 1, 1, 9					
Erodium cicutarium (alfilaria)		NA 40					
Erysimum capitatum (western wallflower)		HO, NA 12, 1					
Eupatorium herbaceum (western throughwort)		NA 34					
Euphorbia spp. (8) (spurge)	PH? 1	HO, NA 36, 1					
Eurotia lanata (winterfat)		HO, NA 1, 1		PH 22			
Evolulus pilosa (evolulus)		NA 39					

	FOOD, BEVERAGE, SMOKING	MEDICINE	CONSTRUCTION FUEL	IMPLEMENTS CEREMONIAL	BASKETS	TEXTILES, CORDAGE, MATTING	DYE, PAINT, TANNING, SOAP
Fallugia paradoxa (Apache plume)		NA 34		HO, NA 36, 34			
Fendlera rupicola (cliff fendlerbush)		HO, NA 12, 1		PH, NA 1,1,			
Forestiera neomexicana (New Mexico olive)		NA 1		HO 36			NA 5
Fragaria spp. (2) (wild strawberry)	NA, UT, SP 1, 1, 6	NA 34					
Gaillardia pinnatifida (blanketflower)		HO, NA 12, 1					
Galium fendleri (bedstraw)		NA 34					
Garrya sp. (silk-tassel)		SP 6		PH 26			
Gaura spp. (3) (gaura)		HO, NA 36, 34					
Gaultheria humifusa (creeping wintergreen)							NA 14
Gayophytum spp.(2) (gayophytum)		NA 1					
Gentiana affinis (pleated gentian)		NA 14					
Geranium spp. (3) (wild geranium)		NA 1					
Gilia spp. (3) (gilia)		NA 1					NA 5
Glycyrrhiza lepidota (wild licorice)		NA, SP 34, 6					
Gnaphalium chilense (everlasting)		NA 34					
Grayia sp. (hop-sage)				PH 26			
Grindelia spp. (2) (gumweed)		NA, UT 1, 9					
Gutierrezia sarothrae (broom snakeweed)		HO, NA, UT 1, 1, 2					
Haplopappus spp. (4) (goldenweed)		HO, NA 36, 1					
Hedeoma drummondii (false pennyroyal)		NA 34					
Hedyotis rubra (bluets)		NA 40					
Helenium hoopesii (orange sneezeweed)		NA 14					NA 1
Helianthella parryi (Parry wood-sunflower)		NA 39					
Helianthus spp. (2) (sunflower)	PH, MO 1, 1	HO, NA 12, 1		PH 23			HO, NA 1, 1
Heliotropium convolvulaceum (bindweed heliotrope)	NA 40						
Heuchera spp. (2) (alumroot)		NA 1					

	FOOD, BEVERAGE, SMOKING	MEDICINE	CONSTRUCTION FUEL	IMPLEMENTS CEREMONIAL	BASKETS	TEXTILES, CORDAGE, MATTING	DYE, PAINT, TANNING, SOAP
Hieracium fendleri (hawkweed)		NA 1					
Hilaria jamesii (galleta)		NA 1		HO 1			
Hoffmanseggia spp. (2) (hog potato)		NA 39					
Holodiscus dumosus (mountain spray)		NA 34					
Humulus americanus (hop)		NA 34					
Hymenopappus spp. (4) (white ragweed)	HO 12	HO, NA 36, 1					HO 12
Hymenoxys spp. (5) (bitterweed)		HO, NA 1					NA 5
Ipomopsis spp. (4) (ipomopsis)		HO, NA 1, 1					HO 12
Iris missouriensis (Rocky Mountain iris)	SP 6	NA 1					NA 14
Iva spp. (2) (marsh-elder)		NA, UT 1, 9					
Juncus sp. (rush)	PH 3	NA 24					
Juniperus deppeana (alligator juniper)	NA 34						
Juniperus osteosperma (Utah juniper)	PH?, MO 1, 1	HO, NA 1, 1	NA, UT 1, 1	NA, UT 1, 1		NA, UT 1, 1	NA 5
Juniperus scopulorum (Rocky Mountain juniper)	UT 7	NA 1		PH 22			
Juniperus sp. (juniper)	PH? 1		PH 1	PH 1		PH 1	
Lactuca serriola (prickly-lettuce)		NA 34					
Lappula spp. (2) (stickseed)		NA 1					
Lathyrus graminifolius (peavine)		NA 39					
Lepidium spp. (3) (peppergrass)	PH 1	NA, SP 1, 1					
Lesquerella spp. (3) (bladderpod)		NA 1					
Leucelene ericoides (white aster)		HO, NA 36, 34					
Ligusticum porteri (osha)		SP 6					
Linanthastrum nuttallii (linanthastrum)		NA 34					
Linum spp. (3) (flax)		HO, NA 36, 1					
Lithospermum spp. (2) (puccoon)		HO, NA 1, 1					
Lomatium orientale (biscuit-root)		NA 14					JE 9

	FOOD, BEVERAGE, SMOKING	MEDICINE	CONSTRUCTION, FUEL	IMPLEMENTS, CEREMONIAL	BASKETS	TEXTILES, CORDAGE, MATTING	DYE, PAINT, TANNING, SOAP
Lonicera spp. (2) (honeysuckle)		NA 1					
Lotus wrightii (deervetch)	NA 1						
Lupinus spp. (6) (lupine)		NA 1					NA 39
Lychnis drummondii (campion)		NA 34					
Lycium pallidum (wolfberry)	PH, HO, NA, SP 13, 1, 1, 6	NA 1					
Lygodesmia spp. (2) (skeleton plant)	HO, NA 1, 1						
Machaeranthera spp. (3) (purple aster)		HO, NA 36, 1					
Malacothrix spp. (2) (desert dandelion)		NA 1					
Malva neglecta (mallow)		NA 24					
Mammillaria sp. (pincushion cactus)	NA 14						
Menadora scabra (rough mendadora)		NA 34					
Mentha arvensis (field mint)		NA 1					
Mentzelia albicaulis (whitestem blazing star)	PH, HO, NA, SP 1, 15, 1, 6	HO, NA 12, 14					
Mentzelia pumila (common stickleaf)	NA, SP 14, 6	HO, NA 36, 1					
Microsteris gracilis (microsteris)		UT 9					
Mimulus eastwoodiae (monkeyflower)		NA 40					
Mirabilis multiflora (four-o'clock)		HO, NA 12, 1					NA 1
Mirabilis oxybaphus (four-o'clock)		NA 1					
Moldavica parviflora (dragonhead)		NA 34					
Monarda spp. (3) (bee-balm)	HO 36	NA 1					
Myosurus spp. (3) (mousetail)		NA 34					
Nama hispidum (nama)		NA 40					
Nicotiana attenuata (coyote tobacco)	PH?, HO, NA, UT, SP 1, 36, 1, 1, 1						
Nicotiana trigonophylla (desert tobacco)	NA, SP 36, 6						
Oenothera spp. (10) (evening-primrose)		HO, NA 36, 1					
Opuntia whipplei (Whipple's cholla)	HO, SP 36, 19						

	FOOD, BEVERAGE, SMOKING	MEDICINE	CONSTRUCTION FUEL	IMPLEMENTS CEREMONIAL	BASKETS	TEXTILES, CORDAGE, MATTING	DYE, PAINT, TANNING, SOAP
Opuntia sp. (cholla)	PH 1						
Opuntia spp. (2) (prickly pear)	PH, HO, NA, SP 1, 36, 24, 1						NA, UT 1, 7
Orobanche fasciculata (broomrape)	NA, SP 40, 6	NA 1					
Orthocarpus purpureo-albus (owlclover)		NA 1					
Oryzopsis hymenoides (Indian ricegrass)	PH, MO 1, 1						
Oxybaphus spp. (4) (desert four-o'clock)		HO, NA 34, 1					
Oxytropis lambertii (Lambert locoweed)	NA 40	NA 40					
Pachystima myrsinites (boxleaf)	NA 1						
Parryella filifolia (dune broom)		HO, NA 36, 1		HO 36	HO, NA 36, 34		HO 36
Parthenocissus inserta (western five-leaved ivy)		NA 1					
Pectis angustifolia (lemoncillo)	PH?, HO 23, 1	NA 14					HO 11
Penstemon spp. (8) (penstemon)		NA 1					
Perezia wrightii (perezia)		NA, SP 1, 6					
Pericome caudata (pericome)		NA 1					
Perideridia sp. (yampa)	UT, SP 31, 6						
Petalostemum spp. (2) (prairie-clover)		NA 20					
Phacelia heterophylla (scorpionweed)	NA 40						
Philadelphus microphyllus (mock-orange)				PH 1			
Phlox spp. (2) (phlox)	NA 40	NA 1					
Phoradendron juniperinum (juniper mistletoe)	HO, NA 36, 1	HO, NA 1, 1					
Phragmites communis (common reed)	PH, SP 1, 6	NA 1	PH, UT 1, 31	PH, HO, UT, SP 1, 36, 1, 19	PH 4		
Phyla cuneifolia (phyla)		NA 40					
Physalis spp. (3) (groundcherry)	PH, HO, NA 1, 36, 20	NA 1					
Physaria newberryi (twin-pod)		HO, NA 15, 39					
Picea spp. (2) (spruce)		NA 1	PH 38				
Pinus edulis (piñón pine)	PH, MO 1, 1	HO, NA 1, 1	PH, NA 1, 14	PH, HO, NA, UT 1, 36, 1, 31			HO, NA, SP 11, 1, 19

	FOOD, BEVERAGE, SMOKING	MEDICINE	CONSTRUCTION, FUEL	IMPLEMENTS, CEREMONIAL	BASKETS	TEXTILES, CORDAGE, MATTING	DYE, PAINT, TANNING, SOAP
Pinus flexilis (limber pine)		NA 1					
Pinus ponderosa (ponderosa pine)		NA 1	PH, MO 1, 1	PH, NA 1, 24			
Plantago spp. (2) (plantain)		NA 1					
Polanisia sp. (clammyweed)	PH? 13						
Poliomintha incana (hoary rosemary-mint)	PH?, HO 23, 1	HO, NA 12, 1					
Polygonum spp. (4) (knotweed)		NA 1					
Populus tremuloides (aspen)	HO, UT 36, 31		HO, NA 36, 14	PH, HO, NA, UT, SP 1, 36, 1, 31, 19			UT 31
Populus spp. (2) (cottonwood)	PH 37		PH 1	PH, HO 1, 12			
Portulaca retusa (notchleaf purslane)	PH, HO, NA, UT 1, 15, 1, 6	NA 40					
Potentilla spp. (4) (cinquefoil)		NA 1					
Prosopis spp. (2) (mesquite)	JI, SP 28, 6			NA 14			
Prunus americana (wild plum)	NA, UT 8, 7						NA 5
Prunus virginiana (chokecherry)	PH, NA, UT, JI 1, 1, 7, 28	NA 1		PH, UT 27, 1			NA, JI 1, 2
Psathyrotes pilifera (psathyrotes)		NA 40					
Pseudocymopterus montanus (mountain parsley)	HO, NA 12, 34	NA 1					NA 5
Pseudotsuga menziesii (Douglas-fir)		NA 1	PH 1	PH 1			
Psilostrophe spp. (2) (paperflower)		NA 1					
Psoralea spp. (3) (scurfpea)	NA, UT 14, 6	NA 1					
Pteridium aquilinum (western bracken)		NA 10			NA 10		
Pterospora andromedea (pinedrops)							NA 5
Purshia tridentata (bitterbrush)		NA, UT 1, 35		NA 14			
Pyrola chlorantha (wintergreen)		NA 40					
Quercus gambelii (Gambel oak)	NA, SP 1, 19			PH, HO, NA 22, 12, 1			NA 1
Quercus spp. (3) (oak)	PH, UT, JI 1, 7, 28		PH 1	PH 1			
Ranunculus spp. (2) (buttercup)		NA 1					

	FOOD, BEVERAGE, SMOKING	MEDICINE	CONSTRUCTION FUEL	IMPLEMENTS CEREMONIAL	BASKETS	TEXTILES, CORDAGE, MATTING	DYE, PAINT, TANNING, SOAP
Ratibida spp. (2) (coneflower)		NA 34					
Rhus glabra (smooth sumac)	SP 6	SP 6					SP 1
Rhus trilobata (threeleaf sumac)	PH, MO 1, 1	HO, NA 1, 1		PH, HO, NA, UT 1, 1, 1, 31	PH, MO 1, 1		HO, NA, JI 1, 1, 2
Ribes spp. (2) (wild currant)	HO, NA 15, 1	NA 1		HO, NA 36, 40			HO 36
Ribes sp. (gooseberry or currant)	PH, UT 1, 1			PH 27			
Rosa woodsii (wild rose)	NA, UT, SP 1, 16, 16	NA 14		UT 31			
Rubus spp. (2) (raspberry, thimbleberry)	NA, UT, SP 8, 1, 6						
Rudbeckia laciniata (brown-eyed susan)		NA 24					
Rumex spp. (3) (wild dock)	NA, SP 14, 19	HO, NA 36, 1					HO, NA, SP 1, 1, 6
Sagittaria cuncata (arrowhead)		NA 14					
Salix spp. (3) (willow)		NA 34	UT 1	PH, NA, UT 1, 1, 1	PH, NA, UT, JI, SP 1, 1, 1, 2, 19	PH 1	UT 1
Salvia carnosa (sage)		HO 36					
Sambucus sp. (elderberry)	UT 7			PH, UT 27, 30			
Sanvitalia abertii (sanvitalia)		NA 1					
Sarcobatus vermiculatus (greasewood)	NA, SP 1, 1	NA 1	PH, HO 1, 36	PH, HO, NA, UT, SP 1, 36, 1, 1, 19			
Scirpus spp. (2) (bulrush)	UT 9	NA 34		PH 23	PH 4	PH 1	
Sclerocactus whipplei (sclerocactus)	PH 18						
Senecio spp. (7) (groundsel)		HO, NA 1, 1		PH 22			
Shepherdia spp. (3) (buffaloberry)	UT, SP 1, 1	NA 1					
Sidalcea neomexicana (prairie mallow)		NA 1					
Silene lacinata (Mexican campion)		NA 1					
Sisymbrium linearifolium (wild mustard)		NA 1					
Smilacina stellata (false Solomon's seal)		NA 34					
Solanum elaeagnifolium (horse-nettle)	NA 1	NA 14					
Solanum jamesii (wild potato)	HO, NA, SP 1, 1, 6						
Solidago spp. (3) (goldenrod)	HO 8	HO, NA 36, 1					HO 11

	FOOD, BEVERAGE, SMOKING	MEDICINE	CONSTRUCTION, FUEL	IMPLEMENTS, CEREMONIAL	BASKETS	TEXTILES, CORDAGE, MATTING	DYE, PAINT, TANNING, SOAP
Sophora sericea (sophora)		NA 39					
Sparganium sp. (bur-reed)	PH? 21						
Sphaeralcea spp. (3) (globe-mallow)	PH?, HO, NA, SP 1, 36, 1, 19	HO, NA, UT 1, 1, 2					
Sporobolus spp. (4) (dropseed)	PH, HO, NA, SP 1, 1, 34, 6	NA 34		PH 23			
Stanleya spp. (2) (desert plume)	HO, NA, SP 1, 1, 1	NA 1					
Stephanomeria pauciflora (wire-lettuce)		NA 34					
Streptanthus cordatus (twistflower)		NA 40					
Suaeda torreyana (Torrey seepweed)	NA 14						
Swertia spp. (3) (deer's ears)		NA 1					
Symphoricarpos spp. (2) (snowberry)	PH 25	NA 40					
Tagetes micrantha (wild marigold)		NA 14					NA 1
Talinum parviflorum (flame flower)		NA 34					
Tetradymia canescens (horsebush)	PH? 17	HO, NA 36, 1					
Thalictrum fendleri (meadow-rue)		NA 39					
Thelesperma spp. (2) (Indian tea)	HO, NA, UT 1, 1, 2	NA 1					HO, NA, JI 1, 14, 2
Thelypodium spp. (2) (wild mustard)		NA 34					
Thermopsis pinetorum (big golden-pea)		NA 34					
Townsendia spp. (3) (Townsend's aster)		NA 1					NA 5
Tradescantia spp. (2) (spiderwort)	HO 12	NA 34					
Tragia nepetaefolia (noseburn)		NA 34					
Triglochin sp. (arrowgrass)		NA 24					
Tripterocalyx wootonii (Wooton sand verbena)		NA 34					
Typha spp. (2) (cattail)	HO, NA, SP 36, 34, 19	NA 1				NA, UT 34, 1	
Urtica gracilis (stinging nettle)		NA 39				UT 7	
Valeriana edulis (thickleaf valerian)	SP 6						
Vancleavea stylosa (vancleavea)		NA 40					

	FOOD, BEVERAGE, SMOKING	MEDICINE	CONSTRUCTION FUEL	IMPLEMENTS CEREMONIAL	BASKETS	TEXTILES, CORDAGE, MATTING	DYE, PAINT, TANNING, SOAP
Verbena spp. (3) (vervain)		NA 1					
Verbesina encelioides (crownbeard)		HO, NA 36, 1					
Veronica spp. (2) (speedwell)		NA 34					
Vicia americana (American vetch)		PH?, NA 21, 34					
Viguiera spp. (3) (goldeneye)	SP 6	NA 34					
Viola nephrophylla (northern bog violet)		NA 34					
Vitis arizonica (canyon grape)	PH, NA, SP 17, 14, 6						
Woodsia mexicana (woodsia)		NA 34					
Wyethia scabra (mulesears)		HO, NA 36, 40					
Yucca angustissima (narrowleaf yucca)	NA 1	HO, NA 1, 1		PH 22	PH, HO 4, 1	PH, NA 22, 1	HO, NA, UT 12, 5, 2
Yucca baccata (banana yucca)	PH, MO 17, 33			PH 1	PH, HO 4, 1	PH 1	HO, NA, JI 1, 1, 2
Yucca sp. (yucca)	PH 1			PH, UT 1, 30	PH 1	PH 1	PH, UT 1, 1
Zigadenus spp. (2) (deathcamus)	NA 40	NA 1					
Zinnia grandiflora (Rocky Mountain zinnia)		NA 1					
TOTAL PLANTS EACH USE	161	423	16	50	11	13	59

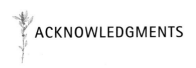 ACKNOWLEDGMENTS

Many people have helped us with this book, some of whom we have met only through their articles, journals, and unpublished reports. Much of the people-plant use information comes from very early written material by those wise people who valued American Indian herbal knowledge and recorded it. For those young colleagues and our contemporaries who are still trying to "get the information out there," we hope we have done well by you in our interpretation of your facts. We accept all responsibility for any errors that might have crept in and hope that they won't be serious ones.

This book is as much about the people of the Four Corners as it is about the useful plants growing there. We were privileged to meet some contemporary natives of this land who graciously shared some of their personal knowledge of the wild plants or who guided us in reconstructing the story of their own people. Among them we are grateful to Rudy Begay of the Chinle Curriculum Center; Veronica Cuthair and Ernest House, who direct the Ute Mountain Tribal Park; Jon Joshevama of the Hopi Cultural Preservation Office; Lydia Pesata, Jicarilla Apache basket weaver; Neomi Red of the Southern Ute Culture Center Museum; and Harry Walters, chairperson for the Center of Diné Studies at the Tsaile Navajo Community College.

With our focus on public parks in the Four Corners country, we relied heavily on park superintendents and their staffs for help during our regular visits, especially for botanical and archaeological information and archival assistance. Individuals who deserve special mention include Dabney Ford, Phil Lopicolo, Joan Mathien, Joyce Raab, Butch Wilson, and Tom Windes of Chaco Culture National Historical Park; Liz Bauer, Marilyn Colyer, Mona Hutchinson, Linda Martin, Will Morris, Donna Reed, and Larry Wiese at Mesa Verde National Park; Anna

Marie Fender and Tara Travis at Canyon de Chelly National Monument; Barry Cooper and Terry Nichels at Aztec Ruins National Monument; LouAnn Jacobson at the Anasazi Heritage Center; Art Hutchinson at Hovenweep National Monument; Veronica Cuthair and Ernest House at Ute Mountain Tribal Park; and Wilson Davis at Monument Valley Navajo Tribal Park. We are proud of these parks and their stewards.

We especially want to thank the museums and other institutions that furthered our cause. The University of New Mexico Herbarium under the direction of Tim Lowrey and Jane Mygatt helped Gail locate plant specimens for her drawings. Assistance in library research and acquiring historical and archival photographs came to Bill from the Museum of New Mexico's Laboratory of Anthropology through Bruce Bernstein, Doty Fugate, Laura Holt, Anita McNeece, Ruth Meria, Willow Powers, Curt Schaafsma, and Louise Stiver; and from the Maxwell Museum through George and Gloria Duck. Karen Adams of the Crow Canyon Archaeological Center shared much ethnobotanical information and was a major reviewer of selected manuscript. Other interviewees who provided valuable insight include Brett Bakker of Native Seeds/SEARCH; Linda Goodman, Janet Spivy, and Mollie Toll of the Museum of New Mexico's Office of Archaeological Studies; and Dave Hafner of the New Mexico Museum of Natural History. Michael J. Gonzales and Glen Kaye of the National Park Service were extremely helpful. Individuals who offered important information or assisted with photography or with personal contacts include J. J. Brody, David Ewing, Judith Phillips, and Bob Swift.

We are indebted to many who provided critical review of portions of the manuscript: Karen Adams, Arthur Harris, Jon Joshevama, Joan Mathien, Will Morris, Harry Walters, Tom Windes, Joe Winter, and Paul Zolbrod. We are especially grateful to Mollie Toll, a friend who cheerfully reviewed most of the text and was always willing to share her ethnobotanical insight and personal observations throughout the entire project.

We are grateful to Blair Clark of the Museum of New Mexico for his new photographs of specimens from the Laboratory of Anthropology collection.

It has once again been a joy to work with the entire staff of the Museum of New Mexico Press. The professional competence of Editorial Director Mary Wachs and Art Director David Skolkin is reflected throughout this book. It was not always easy for them!

Finally, we wish to thank our beloved spouses, Martin Tierney and Vangie Dunmire, for forgiving us the "summer from hell" when we found ourselves still writing, drawing, and photographing with the book due in a month. And then, to add insult to injury, expecting them to be as enthusiastic as we were when we eagerly read excerpts to them at odd times of the night or day. True love was never so tested. Thank you Vangie, thank you Martin.

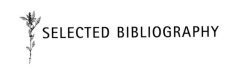

SELECTED BIBLIOGRAPHY

The following references include both works cited in the text and a selection of additional materials researched in the preparation of this publication.

Adams, Karen R.
1980a   Pollen, Parched Seeds and Prehistory: A Pilot Investigation of Prehistoric Plant Remains from Salmon Ruin, a Chacoan Pueblo in Northwestern New Mexico. In *Eastern New Mexico Contributions in Anthropology, Vol. 9.* Eastern New Mexico University, Portales.

1980b   *Pines and Other Conifers from Salmon Ruin, Northwestern New Mexico: Their Identification and Former Role in the Lives of the Ancient People.* Unpublished manuscript.

1993   Carbonized Plant Remains. In *The Duckfoot Site, Vol. 1: Descriptive Archaeology,* ed. by Ricky R. Lightfoot and Mary C. Etzkorn. Occasional Paper No. 3. Crow Canyon Archaeological Center, Cortez, CO.

Adovasio, J. M. and J. D. Gunn
1986   The Antelope House Basketry Industry. In *Archaeological Investigations at Antelope House,* ed. by Don P. Morris. National Park Service, Washington, DC.

Anderson, Edgar
1952   *Plants, Man and Life.* Little, Brown & Co., Boston.

Ayensu, Edward S.
1981   A Worldwide Role for the Healing Powers of Plants. *Smithsonian* 12(8):87–97.

Balick, Michael J. and Paul Alan Cox
1966   *Plants, People and Culture: The Science of Ethnobotany.* Scientific American Library, New York.

Betancourt, Julio L. and Owen K. Davis
1984   Packrat Middens from Canyon de Chelly, Northeastern Arizona: Paleoecological and Archaeological Implications. *Quaternary Research* 21:56–64.

Betancourt, Julio L. and Thomas R. Van Devender
1981   Holocene Vegetation in Chaco Canyon, New Mexico.
Science 214:656–658.

Betancourt, Julio L., Jeffrey S. Dean, and Herbert M. Hull
1986   Prehistoric Long-Distance Transport of Construction
Beams, Chaco Canyon, New Mexico. *American Antiquity*
51(2):370–375.

Betancourt, Julio L., Thomas R. Van Devender, and Paul S. Martin
1990   *Packrat Middens: The Last 40,000 Years of Biotic Change.*
University of Arizona Press, Tucson.

Binford, Lewis R.
1980   Willow Smoke and Dog's Tails: Hunter-Gatherer
Settlement Systems and Archaeological Site Formation. *American
Antiquity* 45(1):4–20.

Bisset, Norman Grainger, ed.
1994   *Herbal Drugs and Phytopharmaceuticals.* Medpharm
Scientific Publishers, Stuttgart; CRC Press, Ann Arbor.

Bohrer, Vorsila L.
1983   New Life from Ashes: The Tale of the Burnt Bush (*Rhus
trilobata*). *Desert Plants* 5:122-124.

1986   Guideposts in Ethnobotany. *Journal of Ethnobiology*
6(1):27–43.

Bradfield, Maitland
1971   The Changing Pattern of Hopi Agriculture. *Royal
Anthropological Institute, Occasional Paper No. 30.* London.

Brew, J. O.
1979   Hopi Prehistory and History to 1850. In *Handbook of North
American Indians, Vol. 9, Southwest,* ed. by Alfonso Ortiz.
Smithsonian Institution, Washington, DC.

Brody, J. J.
1990   *The Anasazi: Ancient Indian People of the American
Southwest.* Rizzoli, New York.

Brown, Kenneth A.
1995   *Four Corners: History, Land, and People of the Desert
Southwest.* HarperCollins, New York.

Brugge, David M.
1983   Navajo History and Prehistory to 1850. In *Handbook of North American Indians, Vol. 10, Southwest,* ed. by Alfonso Ortiz. Smithsonian Institution, Washington, DC.

Bryan, Nonabah G. and Stella Young
1940   *Navajo Native Dyes: Their Preparation and Use.* U.S. Office of Indian Affairs, Washington, DC.

Bryant, Vaughn M., Jr.
1974   The Role of Coprolite Analysis in Archeology. *Bulletin of the Texas Archeological Society.* Austin, TX.

Bye, Robert A.
1972   Ethnobotany of the Southern Paiute Indians in the 1870s. In *Great Basin Cultural Ecology: A Symposium,* ed. by D. Fowler. Desert Research Institute Publications in the Social Sciences, Reno.

Callaway, Donald, Joel Janetski, and Omer C. Stewart
1986   Ute. In *Handbook of North American Indians, Vol. 11, Great Basin,* ed. by Warren L. d'Azevedo. Smithsonian Institution, Washington, DC.

Castetter, Edward F.
1935   *Uncultivated Native Plants Used as Sources of Food.* Ethnobiological Studies in the American Southwest No. 1. University of New Mexico, Albuquerque.

Chamberlin, Ralph V.
1909   Some Plant Names of the Ute Indians. *American Anthropologist* 11:27–40.

Chinle Curriculum Center
1995   *Diné Bikéyahdóó Ch'il Nanise' Altaas'éí: The Purpose and Uses of Plants of Navajoland.* Chinle Unified School District No. 24. Chinle, AZ.

Clary, Karen H.
1984   Anasazi Diet and Subsistence as Revealed by Coprolites from Chaco Canyon. In *Recent Research on Chaco Prehistory,* ed. by W. J. Judge and J. Schelberg. Reports of the Chaco Center No. 8. National Park Service, Albuquerque.

Coe, Sophie D.
1994   *America's First Cuisines.* University of Texas Press, Austin.

Colton, Mary-Russell Ferrell
1965   *Hopi Dyes.* Museum of Northern Arizona, Flagstaff.

Colton, Harold S.
1974   *Hopi Ethnobotany and Archaeological History.* Garland
Publishing, Inc., New York.

Colyer, Marilyn and Linda Martin
1980   *Some Wild Plants of Mesa Verde and Their Uses.*
Mimeograph. Mesa Verde National Park, CO.

Cordell, Linda S.
1984   *Prehistory of the Southwest.* Academic Press, San Diego.

Cruse, Robert R.
1949   A Chemurgic Survey of the Desert Flora in the American
Southwest. *Economic Botany* 3:111–131.

Cully, Anne C.
1985   Pollen Evidence of Past Subsistence and Environment at
Chaco Canyon, New Mexico. In *Environment and Subsistence of
Chaco Canyon, New Mexico,* ed. by Frances Joan Mathien. National
Park Service, Albuquerque.

Cummings, Linda Scott
1993   Anasazi Diet: Variety and Nutritional Analysis. In
Proceedings of the Anasazi Symposium 1991. Mesa Verde Museum
Association, Mesa Verde, CO.

Delaney, Robert W.
1989   *The Ute Mountain Utes.* University of New Mexico Press,
Albuquerque.

Dick-Peddie, William A.
1993   *New Mexico Vegetation: Past, Present and Future.* University
of New Mexico Press, Albuquerque.

Dillingham, Rick et al.
1989   *I Am Here: Two Thousand Years of Southwest Indian Arts and
Culture.* Museum of New Mexico Press, Santa Fe.

Dodgen, Dulce N.
1978   Appendix B: Technical Analysis. In *Wooden Ritual Artifacts
from Chaco Canyon New Mexico: The Chetro Ketl Collection* by R.
Gwinn Vivian, Dulce N. Dodgen, and Gayle H. Hartmann.
University of Arizona Press, Tucson.

Doebley, John F.
1981   Plant Remains Recovered by Floatation from Trash at Salmon Ruin, New Mexico. *The Kiva* 46(3):169–187.

Dunmire, William W. and Gail D. Tierney
1995   *Wild Plants of the Pueblo Province: Exploring Ancient and Enduring Uses.* Museum of New Mexico Press, Santa Fe.

Ebeling, Walter
1986   *Handbook of Indian Foods and Fibers of Arid America.* University of California Press, Berkeley.

Eddington, Patrick and Susan Makov
1995   *Trading Post Guidebook: Where to Find the Trading Posts, Galleries, Auctions, Artists, and Museums of the Four Corners Region.* Northland Publishing, Flagstaff.

Elliott, Michael Lee
1986   *Atlatl Cave and the Late Archaic Period in Chaco Canyon, New Mexico.* Unpublished M.A. thesis, University of New Mexico, Albuquerque.

Elmore, Francis H.
1944   *Ethnobotany of the Navajo.* The University of New Mexico Bulletin with the School of American Research. University of New Mexico Press, Albuquerque.

El-Najjar, Mahmoud Y.
1986   The Biology and Health of the Prehistoric Inhabitants of Canyon de Chelly. In *Archaeological Investigations at Antelope House,* ed. by Don P. Morris. National Park Service, Washington, DC.

Fewkes, J. Walter
1896   A Contribution to Ethnobotany. *American Anthropologist* 9:14–21.

Ford, Richard I., ed.
1978   *The Nature and Status of Ethnobotany.* Anthropological Papers No. 67. Museum of Anthropology, University of Michigan, Ann Arbor.

1981   Gardening and Farming Before A.D. 1000: Patterns of Prehistoric Cultivation North of Mexico. *Journal of Ethnobiology* 1(1): 6–27.

1985   The Processes of Plant Food Production in Prehistoric North America. In *Prehistoric Food Production in North America,* ed. by Richard I. Ford. Anthropological Papers No. 75. Museum of Anthropology, University of Michigan, Ann Arbor.

Fowler, Catherine S.
1986   Subsistence. In *Handbook of North American Indians, Vol.11, Great Basin,* ed. by Warren L. d'Azevedo. Smithsonian Institution, Washington, DC.

Fry, Gary F. and H. Johnson Hall
1986   Human Coprolites. In *Archaeological Investigations at Antelope House,* ed. by Don P. Morris. National Park Service, Washington, DC.

Gasser, Robert E.
1982   Anasazi Diet. In *The Coronado Project Archaeological Investigations. The Specialist's Volume: Biocultural Analyses,* compiled by Robert E. Gasser. Coronado Series 4, Museum of Northern Arizona Research Paper 23, Flagstaff.

Gasser, R. E. and E. C. Adams
1981   Aspects of Deterioration of Plant Remains in Archaeological Sites: The Walpi Archeological Project. *Journal of Ethnobiology* 1:182–192.

Gillespie, William B.
1984   Holocene Climate and Environment of Chaco Canyon. In *Environment and Subsistence of Chaco Canyon, New Mexico,* ed. by Frances Joan Mathien. National Park Service, Albuquerque.

1993   Vertebrate Remains from 29SJ 629. In *The Spadefoot Toad Site: Investigations at 29SJ 629, Chaco Canyon, New Mexico: Artifactual and Biological Analysis, Vol. II,* ed. by Thomas C. Windes. Reports of the Chaco Center No. 12. Branch of Cultural Research, Division of Anthropology, National Park Service, Santa Fe.

Gumerman, George J.
1984   *A View from Black Mesa: The Changing Face of Archaeology.* University of Arizona Press, Tucson and London.

1988   A Historical Perspective on Environment and Culture in Anasazi Country. In *The Anasazi in a Changing Environment,* ed. by George J. Gumerman. Cambridge University Press, Cambridge.

Hall, Robert L. and Arthur E. Dennis
1986   Cultivated and Gathered Plant Foods. In *Archaeological Investigations at Antelope House,* ed. by Don P. Morris. National Park Service, Washington, DC.

Hall, Stephen A.
1988   Prehistoric Vegetation and Environment at Chaco Canyon. *American Antiquity* 53:582–592.

Harrington, H. D.
1972   *Western Edible Wild Plants.* University of New Mexico Press, Albuquerque.

Harris, Arthur H.
1985   *Late Pleistocene Vertebrate Paleoecology of the West.* University of Texas, Austin.

Harris, Marvin
1985   *Good to Eat—Riddles of Food and Culture.* Simon and Schuster, New York.

Hastorf, Christine A. and Virginia S. Popper, eds.
1989   *Current Paleoethnobotany, Analytical Methods and Cultural Interpretations of Archaeological Plant Remains.* University of Chicago Press, Chicago.

Hayes, Alden C.
1964   *The Archaeological Survey of Wetherill Mesa, Mesa Verde National Park, Colorado.* Archaeological Research Series No. 7-A. National Park Service, Government Printing Office, Washington, DC.

Heiser, Charles B., Jr.
1973   *Seed to Civilization.* Harvard University Press, Cambridge.

Hocking, George M.
1955   *A Dictionary of Terms in Pharmacognosy and Other Divisions of Economic Botany.* Charles C. Thomas, Springfield, IL.

1956   Some Plant Materials Used Medicinally and Otherwise by the Navajo Indians in the Chaco Canyon, New Mexico. *El Palacio* 63:146–165.

Holloway, Richard G. and Vaughn M. Bryant, Jr.
1986   New Directions of Palynology in Ethnobotany. *Journal of Ethnobiology* 6(1):47–65.

Jefferson, James, Robert Delaney, and Gregory C. Thompson
1972   *The Southern Utes: A Tribal History.* Southern Ute Tribe, Ignacio, CO.

Johannessen, Sissel and Christine A. Hastorf, eds.
1994   *Corn and Culture in the Prehistoric New World.* Westview Press, Boulder.

Johns, Timothy
1990   *With Bitter Herbs They Shall Eat It.* University of Arizona Press, Tucson.

Jones, Volney H. and Robert E. Fonner
1954   Plant Materials from Sites in the Durango and La Plata Areas, Colorado. In *Basketmaker II Sites Near Durango, Colorado,* by Earl H. Morris and Robert F. Burgh. Carnegie Institute of Washington Publication 604, Washington, DC.

Kearney, Thomas H. and Robert H. Peebles
1960   *Arizona Flora.* University of California Press, Berkeley.

Kelly, Isabel T.
1964   Southern Paiute Ethnography. *University of Utah Anthropological Papers No. 69;* Glen Canyon Series No. 21, University of Utah, Salt Lake City.

Kelly, Isabel T. and Catherine S. Fowler
1986   Southern Paiute. In *Handbook of North American Indians, Vol. 11, Great Basin,* ed. by Warren L. d'Azevedo. Smithsonian Institution, Washington, DC.

Kent, Kate Peck
1983   *Prehistoric Textiles of the Southwest.* School of American Research Press and University of Mexico Press, Albuquerque.

1985   *Navajo Weaving: Three Centuries of Change.* School of American Research Press, Santa Fe.

Kidder, Alfred V.
1924   An Introduction to the Study of Southwestern Archaeology with a Preliminary Account of the Excavations at Pecos. *Papers of the Southwest Expedition 1.* Reprinted in 1962 by Yale University Press, New Haven.

Laise, Steve
1990   Environmental Archaeology: Understanding the

Relationships Between the Ancient Ones and Their Physical World. *Crow Canyon Archaeological Center Newsletter.* Autumn 1990:3–11, Cortez, CO.

Lantz, Edith M., Helen W. Gough, and Mae Martha Johnson
1953   Nutritive Values of Some New Mexico Foods. *New Mexico Experiment Station Bulletin 379,* Las Cruces.

Lekson, Stephen H., Rena Swentzell, and Catherine M. Cameron
1993   *Ancient Land, Ancestral Places: Paul Logsdon in the Pueblo Southwest.* Museum of New Mexico Press, Santa Fe.

Lekson, Stephen H.
1994   Thinking about Chaco. In *Chaco Canyon: A Center and Its World,* Mary Peck et al. Museum of New Mexico Press, Santa Fe.

Lewis, Walter H. and Memory P. F. Elvin-Lewis
1977   *Medical Botany: Plants Affecting Man's Health.* John Wiley & Sons, London.

Litzinger, William Joseph
1979   Ceramic Evidence for the Prehistoric Use of Datura in Mexico and the Southwestern United States. *The Kiva* 44 (2-3): 145–156.

Magers, Pamela C.
1986a   Weaving at Antelope House. In *Archaeological Investigations at Antelope House,* ed. by Don P. Morris. National Park Service, Washington, DC.

1986b   Miscellaneous Wooden and Vegetal Artifacts. In *Archaeological Investigations at Antelope House,* ed. by Don P. Morris. National Park Service, Washington, DC.

Marsh, Charles S.
1982   *People of the Shining Mountains.* Pruett Publishing Co., Boulder.

Martin, Gary J.
1995   *Ethnobotany.* Chapman and Hall, London.

Martin, Paul Schultz
1963   *The Last 10,000 Years: A Fossil Pollen Record of the American Southwest.* University of Arizona Press, Tucson.

Martin, William C. and Charles R. Hutchins
1980   *A Flora of New Mexico.* J. Cramer, West Germany.

Mayes, Vernon O. and Barbara Bayless Lacy
1989   *Nanise' A Navajo Herbal.* Navajo Community College Press, Tsaile, AZ.

Mehringer, Peter J., Jr.
1986   Prehistoric Environments. In *Handbook of North American Indians, Vol. 11, Great Basin.* Smithsonian Institution, Washington, DC.

Milo, Richard G.
1993   Corn Production of Chapin Mesa: Growing Season Variability, Field Rotation, and Settlement Shifts. In *Proceeding of the Anasazi Symposium 1991.* Mesa Verde Museum Association, Mesa Verde, CO.

Minnis, Paul E.
1978   Paleoethnobotanical Indicators of Prehistoric Environmental Disturbances: A Case Study. In *The Nature and Status of Ethnobotany.* Anthropological Papers No. 67. Museum of Anthropology, University of Michigan, Ann Arbor.

1981   Seeds in Archaeological Sites: Sources and Some Interpretive Problems. *American Antiquity* 46:143-152.

1989   Prehistoric Diet in the Northern Southwest: Macroplant Remains from Four-Corners Feces. *American Antiquity* 54:543–563.

Minnis, Paul E. and Richard I. Ford
1977   Appendix C: Analysis of Plant Remains from Chimney Rock Mesa, 1970-1972. In *Archaeological Investigations at Chimney Rock Mesa, 1970-1972,* ed. by Frank W. Eddy. Memoirs of the Colorado Archaeological Society, Boulder.

Moore, Michael
1979   *Medicinal Plants of the Mountain West.* Museum of New Mexico Press, Santa Fe.

1989 *Medicinal Plants of the Desert and Canyon West.* Museum of New Mexico Press, Santa Fe.

Morris, Don P.
1986   Dietary Conclusions. In *Archaeological Investigations at Antelope House,* ed. by Don P. Morris. National Park Service, Washington, DC.

Morris, Earl H.
1919   The Aztec Ruin. *Anthropological Papers of the American Museum of Natural History* 26:7-108.

Nabhan, Gary Paul
1989   *Enduring Seeds: Native American Agriculture and Wild Plant Conservation*. North Point Press, San Francisco.

Nichols, Robert F.
1972   *Wetherill Mesa Excavations: Step House, Mesa Verde National Park, Colorado*. Unpublished manuscript. National Park Service, Mesa Verde, CO.

Opler, Morris E.
1936   A Summary of Jicarilla Apache Culture. *American Anthropologist* 38(2):202-223.

Osborne, Carolyn M.
1965   The Preparation of Yucca Fibers: An Experimental Study. In Contributions of the Wetherill Mesa Archaeological Project, assembled by Douglas Osborne. *Memoirs of the Society for American Archaeology*, No. 19. Salt Lake City.

Peckham, Stewart L.
1990   *From This Earth: The Ancient Art of Pueblo Pottery*. Museum of New Mexico Press, Santa Fe.

Pepper, G.
1920   *Pueblo Bonito*. Anthropological Papers of the American Museum of Natural History No. 27.

Pettit, Jan
1990   *Utes—The Mountain People*. Johnson Publishing Co., Boulder.

Potter, Loren D. and Richard Young
1983   Indicator Plants and Archaeological Sites, Chaco Canyon National Monument. *COAS: New Mexico Archeology and History* 1 (4):19-37.

Roys, Ralph L.
1931   *The Ethno-Botany of the Maya*. Middle American Research Series, Publication No. 2. Tulane University, New Orleans.

Sauer, Carl O.
1952   *Agricultural Origins and Dispersals*. Bowman Memorial Lectures, Series 2. The American Geographical Society, New York.

Schaefer, Jerome
1986   Decorated Ceramics and Unfired Clay Objects. In *Archaeological Investigations at Antelope House*, ed. by Don P. Morris. National Park Service, Washington, DC.

Schmutz, Erwin M. and Lucretia Breazeale Hamilton
1979   *Plants that Poison: An Illustrated Guide for the American Southwest.* Northland Press, Flagstaff.

Schultes, Richard Evans and Albert Hofmann
1979   *Plants of the Gods.* McGraw-Hill, New York.

Schultes, Richard Evans and Siri von Reis, eds.
1995   *Ethnobotany: Evolution of a Discipline.* Dioscorides Press, Portland, Oregon

Schwanitz, Franz
1967   *The Origin of Cultivated Plants.* Harvard University Press, Cambridge.

Scott, Linda J.
1979   Dietary Inferences from Hoy House Coprolites: A Palynological Interpretation. *The Kiva* 44:257–281.

Simmons, Alan H.
1986   New Evidence for the Early Use of Cultigens in the American Southwest. *American Antiquity,* 51:73–88.

Simpson, Ruth DeEtte
1953   *The Hopi Indians.* Southwest Museum Leaflet No. 25. Los Angeles.

Smith, Anne M.
1974   *Ethnography of the Northern Utes.* Papers in Anthropology No. 17. Museum of New Mexico Press, Santa Fe.

Smith, Watson
1952   *Kiva Mural Decorations at Awatovi and Kawaika-a.* Papers of the Peabody Museum of American Archaeology and Ethnology, Vol. 37. Harvard University, Cambridge.

Stewart, Omer C.
1971   *Ethnohistorical Bibliography of the Ute Indians of Colorado,* University of Colorado Study Series in Anthropology No. 18, University of Colorado Press, Boulder.

Stiger, Mark A.
1977   *Anasazi Diet: The Coprolite Evidence.* Unpublished M.A.
thesis, University of Colorado, Boulder.

1979 Mesa Verde Subsistence Patterns from Basketmaker to Pueblo
III. *The Kiva* 44:133–144.

Strutin, Michele
1994   *Chaco: A Cultural Legacy.* Southwest Parks and Monuments
Association, Tucson.

Thompson, Ian
1993   *The Towers of Hovenweep.* Mesa Verde Museum
Association, Mesa Verde, CO.

Tierney, Gail D.
1976   Of Pots and Plants. *El Palacio* 82(3):48–52.

1977   Plants for the Dyepot. *El Palacio* 83(3):28–35.

Tiller, Veronica E. Velarde
1982   *The Jicarilla Apache Tribe: A History.* University of Nebraska
Press, Lincoln and London.

1983   Jicarilla Apache. In *Handbook of North American Indians,
Vol. 10, Southwest,* ed. by Alfonso Ortiz. Smithsonian Institution,
Washington, DC.

Toll, Mollie S.
1983   Changing Patterns of Plant Utilization for Food and
Fuel: Evidence from Floatation and Macrobotanical Remains. In
*Economy and Interaction Along the Lower Chaco River: The Navajo
Mine Archeological Program, Mining Area III, San Juan County, New
Mexico,* ed. by Patrick Hogan and Joseph C. Winter. Office of
Contract Archeology and The Maxwell Museum of Anthropology,
University of New Mexico, Albuquerque.

1985   An Overview of Chaco Canyon Macrobotanical Materials
and Analysis to Date. In *Environment and Subsistence of Chaco
Canyon, New Mexico,* ed. by Frances Joan Mathien. National Park
Service, Albuquerque.

1993   Flotation and Macro-botanical Analysis at 29SJ 629. In
*The Spadefoot Toad Site: Investigations at 29SJ 629 Chaco Canyon,
New Mexico: Artifactual and Biological Analysis, Vol. II,* ed. by Thomas

C. Windes. Reports of the Chaco Center No. 12. Branch of
Cultural Research, National Park Service, Santa Fe.

Tyler, S. Lyman
1964   *The Ute People: A Bibliographical Checklist.* Institute of
American Indian Studies. Brigham Young University, Provo.

Tyler, Varro E., Lynn R. Brady, and James E. Robbers
1976   *Pharmacognosy,* 7th ed. Lee and Febiger, Philadelphia.

Van West, Carla R.
1993   Reconstructing Prehistoric Climatic Variability and
Agricultural Production in Southwestern Colorado, A.D. 901–1300:
A GIS Approach. In *Proceedings of the Anasazi Symposium 1991,*
Mesa Verde Museum Association, Mesa Verde, Colorado.

Vestal, Paul A.
1952   Ethnobotany of the Ramah Navaho. *Papers of the Peabody
Museum of American Archaeology and Ethnology* 40(4), Harvard
University, Cambridge.

Vines, Robert I.
1960   *Trees, Shrubs, and Woody Vines of the Southwest.* University
of Texas Press, Austin.

Vivian, R. Gwinn
1990   *The Chacoan Prehistory of the San Juan Basin.* Academic
Press, San Diego.

Vogel, Virgil J.
1970   *American Indian Medicine.* University of Oklahoma Press,
Norman.

Welsh, Stanley L., N. Duane Atwood, Sherel Goodrich, and Larry
C. Higgins, eds.
1987   *A Utah Flora.* Great Basin Naturalist Memoirs No. 9.
Brigham Young University, Provo.

Wheeler, Elizabeth M.
1994   *Mother Earth's Mercantile: Plants of the Four Corners Area
and Their Uses Through Time.* Crow Canyon Archaeological Center,
Cortez, CO.

Whiting, Alfred F.
1939   Ethnobotany of the Hopi. *Museum of Northern Arizona
Bulletin 15.* Flagstaff, AZ.

Williams-Dean, Glenna
1986   Pollen Analysis of Human Coprolites. In *Archaeological Investigations at Antelope House,* ed. by Don P. Morris. National Park Service, Washington, DC.

Williams, Terry Tempest
1983   *Pieces of White Shell—A Journey to Navajoland.* University of New Mexico Press, Albuquerque.

Willink, Roseann S. and Paul G. Zolbrod
1996   *Weaving a World: Textiles and the Navajo Way of Seeing.* Museum of New Mexico Press, Santa Fe.

Windes, Thomas C. and Dabney Ford
1996   The Chaco Wood Project: The Chronometric Reappraisal of Pueblo Bonito. *American Antiquity* 61(2):295-310.

Winter, Joseph C.
1974   *Aboriginal Agriculture in the Southwest and Great Basin.* Unpublished Ph.D. dissertation, Anthropology Department, University of Utah, Salt Lake City.

Winter, Joseph C. and William J. Litzinger
1976   Floral Indicators of Farm Fields. In *Hovenweep 1975,* ed. by Joseph C. Winter. Archaeological Report No. 2. Department of Anthropology, San Jose State University, San Jose.

Worcester, Donald E.
1979   *The Apaches: Eagles of the Southwest.* University of Oklahoma Press, Norman and London.

Wright, Barton
1979   *Hopi Material Culture.* Northland Press, Flagstaff.

Wyman, Leland C. and Stuart K. Harris
1941   Navajo Indian Medical Ethnobotany. *University of New Mexico Bulletin, Anthropological Series* 3(5), Albuquerque.

1951   The Ethnobotany of the Kayenta Navaho: An Analysis of the John and Louisa Wetherill Ethnobotanical Collection. *University of New Mexico Publications in Biology* 5:1–66, Albuquerque.

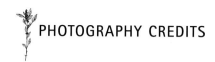

PHOTOGRAPHY CREDITS

All botanical line illustrations by Gail D. Tierney. All photographs by William W. Dunmire except as noted below.

Pg. 25: National Park Service photo, Mesa Verde National Park. Pg. 31, bottom: National Park Service Photo Archives, Western Archeological and Conservation Center. Pg. 31, top: National Park Service Photo Archives, Western Archeological and Conservation Center. Pg. 37: photo by J. Imhof, Maxwell Museum Photo Archives, neg. no. 61.14.151. Pg. 69: photo by Milton Snow, Maxwell Museum Photo Archives, neg. no. 87.44.159. Pg. 40: Maxwell Museum Photo Archives, neg. no. 87.45.201. Pg. 43: Southwest Museum and Maxwell Museum Photo Archives, neg. no. 92.1.15. Pg. 52: Maxwell Museum Photo Archives, neg. no. 92.1.937. Pg. 54: Museum of New Mexico photo, neg. no. 41807. Pg. 56: photo by Douglas Kahn, School of American Research Collection in Museum of New Mexico, cat. no. 23488/12. Pg. 61, top: photo by Milton Snow, Maxwell Museum Photo Archives, neg. no. 87.45.173. Pg. 61, bottom: photo by Milton Snow, Maxwell Museum Photo Archives, neg. no. 87.44.169. Pg. 74: National Park Service, Chaco Culture National Historical Park Museum Collection (Dunmire photo). Pg. 82: National Park Service, Chaco Culture National Historical Park Museum Collection Archives. Pg. 85, top: photo by Blair Clark, Museum of Indian Arts and Culture/Laboratory of Anthropology, cat. no. 53697/12. Pg. 85, bottom: National Park Service, Chaco Culture National Historical Park Museum Collection Archives. Pg. 86: National Park Service Photo Archives, Western Archeological and Conservation Center. Pg. 88: photo by Douglas Kahn, School of American Research Collection in Museum of New Mexico, cat. no. 1729/12. Pg. 90: National Park Service, Mesa Verde National Park Museum Collection (Dunmire photo). Pg. 91: National Park Service, Mesa Verde National Park Museum Collection (Dunmire photo). Pg. 92: photo by Blair Clark, School of American Research Collections in the Museum of New Mexico, cat. no. 9941/12. Pg. 93: National Park Service Photo Archives, Western Archeological and Conservation Center. Pg. 97, top: photo by Mary Peck, Museum of Indian Arts and Culture, Santa Fe, NM, cat. no. 2514/11. Pg. 97, bottom: photo by Mary Peck, Museum of Indian Arts and Culture, Santa Fe, NM; L: cat. no. 19622/11, R: cat. no. 19621/11. Pg. 99: photo by Douglas Kahn, School of American Research Collection in Museum of New Mexico, cat. no. 1131/12. Pg. 102: photo by Steve Lekson, National Park Service, Chaco Culture National Historical Park Museum Collection Archives, neg. no. 14448. Pg. 111: Crow Canyon Archaeological Center Photo Archives. Pg. 112: photo by Blair Clark. Pg. 201: photo by Gail D. Tierney. Pg. 244: photo by Blair Clark, Museum of Indian Arts and Culture/Laboratory of Anthropology, cat. no. 21737/11.

INDEX

ABOUT THE AUTHORS

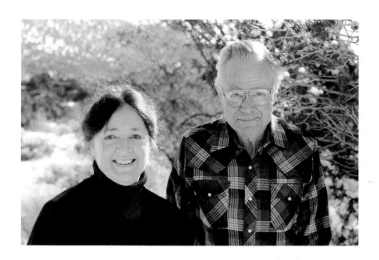

GRADUATE OF the University of California, Berkeley, with degrees in wildlife management and zoology, Bill Dunmire served twenty-eight years in the National Park Service, mostly as a naturalist in a number of parks including Yellowstone and Yosemite. For several years he was a biologist with The Nature Conservancy. A professional nature photographer and author of numerous natural history publications, including, with Gail Tierney, *Wild Plants of the Pueblo Province* (MNMP 1995), Bill lives with his wife, Vangie, in Placitas, New Mexico.

GAIL D. TIERNEY was trained in anthropology, paleoecology, and botany at the University of New Mexico. Over the past thirty years she has been employed as staff or consultant at the Laboratory of Anthropology, Museum of New Mexico, Los Alamos National Laboratory, and other technical or teaching institutions in New Mexico. Author or coauthor of numerous technical reports, popular articles, and three books, she has received several awards for excellence in the writing of "readable science." Gail lives with her husband, Martin, in Santa Fe, New Mexico.